BARE MINIMUM
Dinners

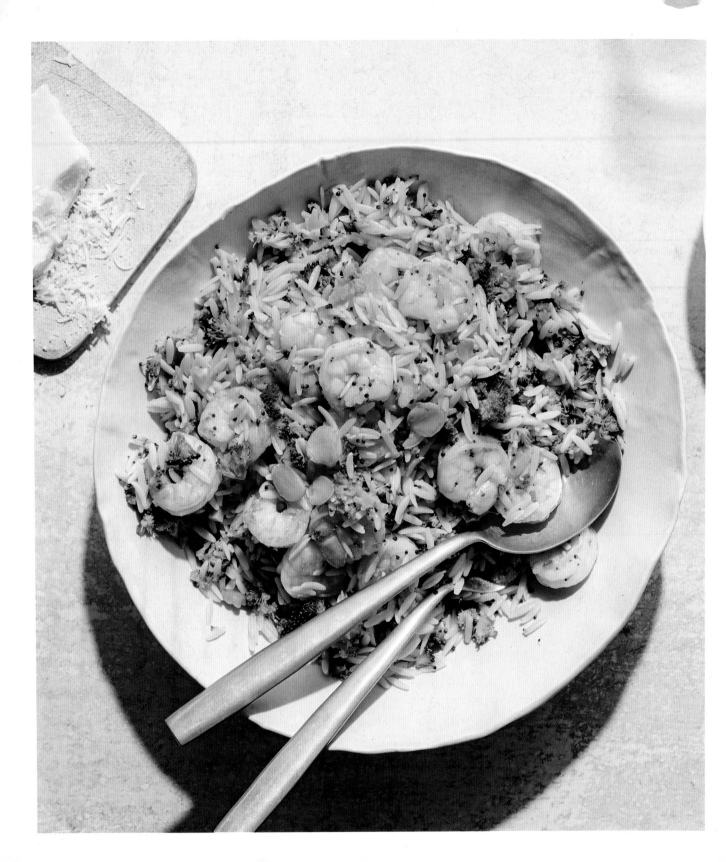

BARE MINIMUM
Dinners

Recipes and Strategies for *Doing Less* in the Kitchen

JENNA HELWIG

HOUGHTON MIFFLIN HARCOURT · BOSTON NEW YORK · 2021

To Dave and Rosen,

My favorite dinner companions

For information about permission to reproduce selections from this book, write to trade.permissions@hmhco.com or to Permissions, Houghton Mifflin Harcourt Publishing Company, 3 Park Avenue, 19th Floor, New York, New York 10016.

hmhbooks.com

Library of Congress Cataloging-in-Publication Data is available.

ISBN 978-0-358-434719 (print)

ISBN 978-0-358-43546-4 (ebook)

Book design by Melissa Lotfy

Printed in China

SCP 10 9 8 7 6 5 4 3 2 1

Contents

3. BARE MINIMUM INGREDIENTS 67
Recipes with Seven Ingredients (or Less)

4. BARE MINIMUM CLEANUP 111
Dinners That Come Together in a Single Pot or Pan

5. BARE MINIMUM HANDS-ON TIME   157

Recipes for the Instant Pot or Slow Cooker

6. BARE MINIMUM SIDES   191

Easy Add-Ons to Round Out Dinner

Acknowledgments

Sharon Bowers, I raise my Negroni glass to you! Cheers to another project together, and thank you for always being in my corner.

To my editor, Stephanie Fletcher, thank you for your faith in me and in the concept of this book. I am so grateful for your guidance. And to the amazing team at HMH, including Rebecca Springer, Bridget Nocera, Samantha Simon, Jacqueline Quirk, and Kevin Watt; working with you is a true pleasure. Melissa Lotfy, thank you for your creative vision and design expertise.

I am blown away by the beauty of the book you're holding in your hands. Credit goes to the photography dream team: Linda Xiao, Maeve Sheridan, and Monica Pierini, who powered through six days of shooting with energy, enthusiasm, and smiles under face masks. Thank you for caring so much about *Bare Minimum Dinners!*

Suzy Scherr, you are a bona fide slow cooker genius, and I'm so appreciative. Renae Wilson, thank you for your meticulous recipe testing and friendship.

The inspiration for this book came from my close friends, the (mostly) women who hustle so hard to feed themselves and the people they love on a daily basis. Cooking dinner most nights is a wonderful thing, but it isn't easy. My friends—consider this book a small thank-you for your enduring love and support. Grace Bastidas, Audrey Bellezza, Heather Date, Allison Graham, Emily Harding, Jessica Winchell Morsa, Nicole Page, Felicity Rowe, Danielle Wilkie, and Zoran Zgonc—you are all in my heart.

Laura Fenton, it's so fun to have you as a companion on this book-writing adventure! Thanks for keeping me accountable.

Thank you to my friends and colleagues at *Real Simple*, *Parents*, and *Health*, especially Liz Vaccariello, who gave me my dream job, and Ananda Eidelstein, with whom it is my true delight to work with every day. Thank you also to Steve Engel and Heidi Reavis; I'm so happy to still be part of the Engel Entertainment "family" after all these years.

Speaking of family—Andy and Linda Helwig, David and China Helwig, Cole, Tasha, and Daphne, I wish I could have dinner with you more often. I love you, and I miss you.

And to my regular dinner companions, Dave and Rosen, thank you for your patience with my experiments, your good humor when things don't go exactly as planned, your enthusiastic appetites, and your unflagging support. You are my everythings.

Introduction

I have spent much of my career urging people to do more in the kitchen—often with the goal of making weeknight dinners less stressful. I've touted weekend meal prep sessions, carefully curated pantries, big batches of dinners for the freezer, homemade marinara sauce, and DIY pizza crust, all with the goal of serving delicious, healthy-ish homemade meals most nights of the week.

I wasn't wrong! And yet...

As my life has become ever busier and my friends' lives have gotten more hectic, and as I've heard from readers and the fans of my previous books, I've had a change of heart. My goal is still the same: more cooking at home for yummy, nourishing dinners. But my strategy has changed.

I realized that instead of doing more, we should all strive to do *less* in the kitchen, to spend less time shopping, cooking, and cleaning up. Of course, this doesn't mean that there won't be special meals or even weekend dinners where we spend an hour or three in the kitchen (and I confess, that's one of my favorite ways to pass the time... when I have the time).

But on a daily basis, life is just too busy—and the truth is, most people (probably you and me included) *would rather be doing something else.*

And while there's no shame in outsourcing dinner occasionally (trust me, I feel no shame), homemade is still the goal, for a whole host of reasons, including:

- Unless you're eating truffles and fancy cheeses every night or, conversely, eating only at fast food joints, home-cooked meals are usually less expensive than restaurant food.

- It's also healthier. The recipes in this book weren't created to fit into any rigid nutritional parameters, but chances are they'll have less sodium, less saturated fat, and more real, whole ingredients than most delivery or takeout food.

- You know exactly what's in your food. Even if you use a jar of store-bought sauce in a meal, you'll be able to see the ingredient list and make choices about what goes into your dinner. This is especially helpful if you or someone in your family has a dietary restriction or food allergy.

So instead of stressing out about dinner, I propose that to feed our families happily, we strive to simply skate by. This cookbook gives you permission to take smart supermarket shortcuts, to skip the mile-long ingredient list, to just say no to pre-prepping homemade sauces, to—gasp!—omit the garnish. In this book, we do the bare minimum, and it tastes delicious.

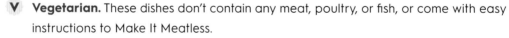

About the Icons

Many of the recipes in this book are marked with one of these two symbols:

V **Vegetarian.** These dishes don't contain any meat, poultry, or fish, or come with easy instructions to Make It Meatless.

✪ **These are the MVPs.** In a word, these recipes are gold. They may show up in any of the main dish chapters, and they deliver on time, ingredients, and equipment, meaning they require 30 minutes or less, include seven ingredients or less, *and* come together in a single pot or pan.

HOW TO USE THIS BOOK

Each chapter addresses a specific dinnertime pain point, be it cook time, ingredients, cleanup, hands-on time, or how to round out a meal. All of them feature recipes that are an easy lift.

Chapter 1 will get you set up for supper success. From recommended kitchen gear to workhorse pantry items, being prepared will make cooking even easier.

Chapter 2 is all about time. Have you ever started to make a meal that promised to be on the table in a half hour only to discover that you needed 15 minutes of ingredient prep to get started? Me too. The recipes in this chapter are the real deal. Many use smart supermarket short-cuts; all of them get delicious food in your family's bellies fast. Because when it comes down to it, most of us have a need for speed on weeknights (and some weekend evenings, too, of course). Whether you're opening the fridge after a commute or trying to help with homework while stirring a pot on the stove, the recipes in this chapter will get a satisfying meal on the table fast.

Chapter 3 cuts to the chase with recipes that use seven ingredients—or less. At the end of a long day, nothing is more daunting than an ingredient list that goes on . . . and on. These recipes won't let you down. They're simple and streamlined and require at most seven ingredients, *including* salt, pepper, and olive oil. In this chapter you'll use items like spice blends and high-quality jarred sauces to get a lot of bang for your ingredient buck. You'll often see olive oil used two ways, as a cooking medium and a finisher. Many recipes include a "Dress It Up" option in case you want to add some visual appeal and an extra punch of flavor to dinner, but these are by no means required.

Chapter 4 streamlines cleanup. Often, what seems so daunting about cooking is the pile of dirty dishes waiting when you're done. These recipes require a single pot, sheet pan, or skillet for easy cleanup.

Chapter 5 lets you set it and forget it. This chapter features Instant Pot and slow cooker meals, each requiring minimal active time—and no additional stove-top browning or broiling in the oven.

Chapter 6 rounds it all out. One of my non-negotiable dinner rules (see page 23) is that the meal must include a vegetable in some shape or form. Often it's part of the main dish, but sometimes you need an easy add-on. Other times you need a little starchy bulk to give supper staying power. These recipes are super-easy ideas for salads, grains, and vegetable sides.

THE RECIPES

The dinners in this book are a mix of longtime family favorites, new discoveries, and adapted versions of friends' bare minimum dinners. I love big flavors and am always excited to incorporate a sauce or a technique or a seasoning from one of the world's great cuisines. So many of these recipes are a little bit something . . . a little bit Korean, a little bit Indian, a little bit Italian, or a little bit Mexican. What these recipes *aren't* is authentic. They're a mishmash of flavors and techniques and a reflection of the culinary variety my family and I crave.

About half of the recipes are vegetarian or pescatarian (meaning no meat or poultry, but some fish) because that is how we eat most nights at my house. But, don't worry, there are plenty of chicken, beef, and pork recipes here too for meat lovers (of which I am unabashedly one).

Most of the recipes serve four people, but some a little more or a little less, and I've included cooking, ingredient, and equipment tips throughout to help make the path from "I'm hungry" to "Let's eat" a little smoother.

Many of the recipes also include these suggestions:

Dress It Up

My time in the magazine business, where every recipe has a photo, has trained me to always think about how a dish will look. By contrast, when cooking a bare minimum dinner at home, looks are not paramount; ease and flavor are. Sometimes, though, it's simple to zhuzh up the look of a dish with a sprinkle of chopped herbs or a dusting of grated cheese. You don't need them, but if you happen to have the cilantro or sesame seeds (or Parm or hot sauce) on hand, go for it! Your dinner will be prettier and boast an extra layer of flavor.

Make It Meatless

Some of the recipes in this book have just a little meat for flavoring and can easily be made without it. In others, you can substitute tofu or eggs for the meat.

Make It Meaty

Conversely, these are vegetarian recipes where it's very easy to add a little animal protein for extra flavor and to satisfy any carnivores at the table. Often there's the option to include meat in only part of the meal for maximum flexibility.

MY COOKING MANTRA

It's going to be fine.

Really. If you don't have a specific ingredient, leave it out or substitute the closest thing you have. Want to use ground turkey instead of ground beef or spinach instead of kale? Go for it! Very rarely will your dinner be ruined beyond all eating. In a pinch, drizzle on some olive oil, spritz with lemon, and sprinkle with salt. Or just be liberal with the hot sauce. It may not be the best thing you've ever cooked, but it's just one dinner. Trust me, I've made my share of just okay dinners and even a few that were true disasters. But, we survived, laughed about it, and didn't starve to death. (There's always PB&J in a pinch.)

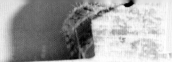

YOUR SETUP

EQUIPMENT

While bare minimum dinners *can* be prepared with bare minimum kitchen tools, you'll find that your cooking life goes more smoothly with the right tool for the job. Here are the essentials.

Pots and Pans

- 5- to 8-quart stockpot or Dutch oven with lid
- 3- to 4-quart pot with lid
- 12- to 14-inch cast-iron or stainless steel skillet or sauté pan
- 10-inch oven-safe, nonstick skillet—Having at least one nonstick skillet is tremendously helpful for cooking eggs and fish, which I find almost impossible to cook properly in stainless. (Tofu and fried rice also prefer nonstick, but are manageable in cast-iron.)

Replace it as soon as it gets scratched or loses its nonstickiness, which will happen. Thankfully, affordably priced nonstick is easy to find.
- 8-inch skillet
- Roasting pan
- 13 × 9-inch baking dish
- 8 × 8-inch baking dish
- Large rimmed baking sheet (aka half-sheet pan)

Prep Pieces

- Large cutting board—Your cutting board is your meal prep home base. Please don't try to make dinner on a small or even medium-sized board. Ingredients will fall off as you chop, and you'll feel crowded and disorganized. Invest in a board that's at least 18 × 12 inches. It can be thick plastic or wood. Avoid boards made of composite materials, since they can dull knives more quickly. Place a damp paper towel or thin dish towel under your board to keep it from slipping on the counter while you work.

- Small or medium-sized cutting board—This is handy for cutting a lemon or grating some cheese without having to wash the big board.
- Set of mixing bowls—Plastic, glass, or ceramic are all fine.
- Large colander
- Handheld strainer
- Instant Pot and/or slow cooker—I use both regularly, but if you're going to get only one, I recommend the Instant Pot or other multicooker. I find it more versatile and absolutely love that you can sauté ingredients in the same pot that the food

is ultimately cooked in. It makes a huge difference in convenience and flavor.
- Salad spinner—My family eats a lot of salads and other leafy greens. Without a salad spinner (I like Zyliss brand), I would probably give up or resort to buying plastic clamshells. See page 195 for how to clean greens.
- 2- and 4-cup liquid measuring cups
- Set of dry measuring cups
- Set of measuring spoons
- Blender—Since I don't think bare minimum dinners should require blending, only one recipe in this book calls for it. You might already have a countertop blender for making smoothies, but an immersion model lets you do the job right in the cooking pot. It's practically effortless, and there's no blender jar to wash.

Handheld Tools

- Sharp chef's knife—Possibly the most essential tool in your kitchen; choose a knife with at least a 6-inch blade for efficient chopping. And keeping your knife sharp is key for faster and more effortless cutting. A dull knife is actually more dangerous since it slips more easily.
- Paring knife
- Large serrated knife for bread and big cuts of meat
- Citrus juicer
- Microplane or other wand-style grater
- Box grater
- 2 silicone spatulas
- 2 wooden spoons
- 1 small spatula
- 2 large spatulas and/or fish spatulas—I love a thin, slatted fish spatula for so much more than fish. It's a crackerjack cookie lifter, cutlet turner, and pot scraper, should you find that necessary. Make sure one spatula is silicone or plastic for use on your nonstick pan.
- Ladle
- Whisk
- 2 sets of tongs
- Instant-read thermometer—This is crucial for cooking meatballs, pork, and chicken to a safe temperature.
- Can opener
- Vegetable peeler—I prefer a sturdy Y-shaped peeler for maximum control.

What's Not on This List

None of the recipes in this book require a food processor, but I'd still encourage you to get one to further simplify your kitchen life. You can use it to make pie crusts and pizza doughs, pestos and dips, not to mention vegetable purées and energy balls. It is one of my most-used pieces of kitchen equipment, just not on a busy weeknight.

THE BARE MINIMUM PANTRY

Open my cabinets and you will see that my pantry is anything but "bare minimum." I am a bit of a food collector, convinced that I'll find a use for that second bag of shredded coconut and small can of pickled jalapeños. And usually I do! But, for weeknight dinners, here are the essentials.

Fats and Vinegars

- **Extra virgin olive oil** I use this for 80 percent (or more) of my cooking. I typically buy California Olive Ranch, but there are many good brands on the market at all price points. Find one you like; that's all that matters.

- **Coconut oil** I love the tropical aroma of coconut and the almost sweet flavor it brings to recipes. Remember that when you cook with coconut oil, you'll likely taste it, so make sure that's a flavor you want in your recipe.

- **Neutral-tasting oil** I reach for this when I don't want the fat I'm using to bring any flavor to the dish. I usually have canola oil on hand, but sometimes grapeseed, sunflower, or safflower.

- **Toasted sesame oil** This is a staple when it comes to adding a warm note to many dishes, especially those with East Asian flavors.

- **Unsalted butter** I keep a few sticks in the fridge at all times, and an extra box or two in the freezer. I never want to be out of butter! I rarely use it to start a dish, but often to finish one.

- **Red wine vinegar** This is my go-to for many salad dressings, and I also add a dash to soups to balance the flavors.

- **Rice vinegar** Essential for many East Asian dishes. It's one of the least acidic vinegars, so I sometimes use it in salad dressings for a milder bite.

- **Apple cider vinegar** A versatile vinegar, ACV is my choice for finishing bean soups, in coleslaw, and anything barbecue-related.

It's rare that the type of vinegar you use will make or break your dish. If you don't have the variety a recipe calls for, just use what's in your pantry.

All the Noodles

I am thankful for many things in life, and one of them is pasta. Not only is a box of regular old dried pasta budget-friendly, it cooks quickly, is surprisingly nutritious (4 ounces of regular semolina pasta contains 14 grams of protein and 4 grams of fiber; whole-grain has 16 grams of protein and 14 grams of fiber), and makes dinner something to look forward to. It's also a great vehicle for vegetables and incredibly versatile. I'm not saying we should all eat pasta every night (although if you twisted my arm I could probably be convinced), but I long ago gave up any compunction about enjoying it on a regular basis.

My favorite mainstream brand of dried pasta is De Cecco, but I will occasionally splurge on a fancy artisanal brand for an even dreamier texture. Here's what I keep around:

- **Short pasta shapes** Penne or rigatoni and orecchiette
- **Orzo** Great for salads and soups
- **Long pasta** Spaghetti or fettucine; I also love egg-based pappardelle
- **Stuffed pasta** Ravioli and tortellini, either refrigerated or frozen (I like Rana brand for refrigerated)
- **Soba noodles** These cook in only a few minutes and are seriously slurpable with a simple peanut or tahini sauce. Or just drizzle them with toasted sesame oil and soy sauce and top with sliced raw veggies. Most grocery store brands of soba are made from a combination of wheat and buckwheat flours, giving them a nutty taste and texture.

Whole Grains, Rice, and Dried Beans

By far, my favorite whole grain is farro, a chewy grain that cooks in under 20 minutes (if you buy a semi-pearled or pearled variety, often labeled *farro perlato*). Farro retains its shape and bite in soups and salads and offers a tasty bed of starch when you need one. I also enjoy the heft of wheatberries, but they take nearly an hour to cook on the stove-top. So I generally save these for cooking in the Instant Pot.

A pot of white rice for four people comes together in under 25 minutes on the stove-top, making it a regular in my dinner rotation. I usually buy an American-grown basmati or jasmine variety and just follow the directions on the package. If I am thinking ahead, I make a double batch and refrigerate or freeze half for fried rice later in the week. (You can cook the rice on the stove-top directly from frozen. It becomes crisp and delicious.)

Brown rice packs a heftier nutritional punch than more-refined white. But, since it takes significantly longer to cook on the stove-top—and somehow I find that preparation trickier—I always make it in the Instant Pot. (Combine 2 cups brown rice, 2 cups water, and ½ teaspoon kosher salt in the Instant Pot. Cook on high pressure for 20 minutes, then let the pressure release naturally for 10 minutes.)

Speaking of the Instant Pot, before I got one, I would work up the ambition to cook dried beans maybe once or twice a year, dutifully remembering to soak the beans ahead of time. But now, thanks to my multicooker, I prepare beans with no forethought at all, tossing them into the appliance with some water, salt, and little else. Served with lashings of olive oil and a dusting of Parm, they're deeply satisfying. All this to say, keep your pantry stocked with a variety of dried beans!

Canned Goods

I start to panic a little if I am without cans of crushed tomatoes, tomato paste, and beans (pinto, black, cannellini, and chickpeas). It's also nice to have a can or two of whole plum tomatoes and diced tomatoes on hand. I like Muir Glen for tomato products and am not picky about canned beans. Amy's brand of refried beans are a ticket to big flavor fast.

Nuts, Seeds, and Dried Fruit

Nuts add flavor, texture, and nutrition to all sorts of recipes. I often lean on them for an extra hit of protein when I'm making meatless meals. Walnuts are my go-to; they're less expensive than almonds and boast more brain-boosting omega-3s than any other tree nut. When I need toasted walnuts for a recipe, I'll toast the whole bag and store whatever I'm not using right away, being sure to label them "toasted." We go through nuts pretty quickly, so I keep them in the pantry; for longer shelf life you can store toasted or untoasted nuts in the freezer. I also keep almonds and pistachios around for snacking and some recipes.

Sesame seeds and pepitas (hulled pumpkin seeds) add nutrition, flavor, texture, and eye appeal to a recipe. Toast them for top flavor.

I am one of those eaters who enjoys a little sweet in my savory, so I often reach for raisins, dried figs, dried cherries, or dates to add a burst of flavor to stews and salads.

To toast nuts or seeds, spread them in a single layer on a rimmed baking sheet. Bake in a 350°F oven or toaster oven until lightly golden and fragrant, 5 to 10 minutes. Keep a close eye on them since they can burn quickly, especially tiny sesame seeds. If you need only a small amount of seeds, you can toast them on the stove-top. Place them in a small skillet and cook over medium heat, stirring frequently, until lightly golden, usually less than 5 minutes. Remove them from the pan immediately as they can go from browned to burnt very quickly.

Shortcuts

You will see that many of the recipes in this book rely on a store-bought sauce or condiment, and even the occasional boxed mix and fun frozen vegetable (I'm looking at you, sweet potato fries). While I love making many staples from scratch, I've come to appreciate the ease of a jar of delicious marinara sauce or package of cheese- and potato-stuffed pierogi, especially when I'm trying to get dinner on the table in under a half hour and didn't have time over the weekend to prep my own pesto, say. Here are some of the store-bought shortcuts I am grateful for, along with my preferred brands. I'm sharing the brand information so you can look for them if you don't have a favorite of your own. If you do, stick with that!

Marinara sauce As you will see, marinara makes frequent appearances in my meals; it's so much more versatile than just as a pasta sauce. I used to make my own all the time, but now I spring for Rao's. It's pricey but worth the splurge for me. If you prefer to buy another brand, look for one without added sugar.

Enchilada sauce A good homemade enchilada sauce usually involves toasting chiles, blending, and then cooking. It's a labor of love that rewards you with every flavorful bite. But for quick dinners, I buy Frontera.

Pesto I love to make my own pesto in the summer, often adding blanched baby spinach or parsley to the basil to keep the mixture green.

I freeze several servings but usually run out by November. Since a good pesto can perk up so many dishes, I rely on store-bought until fragrant basil comes back into season. Skip the shelf-stable jars—neither their flavor nor their color will be vibrant—in favor of refrigerated brands. I recently discovered Gotham Greens pesto, and I'm now rarely without it. Buitoni also makes a solid version.

Indian simmer sauce To be clear, this is not the most authentic path to Indian-inspired dishes, but tikka masala and other Indian sauces are clutch when it comes to quickly adding big flavor to chicken and tofu. My two favorite brands are Maya Kaimal and Masala Mama.

Dried Breadcrumbs

Panko (Japanese-style breadcrumbs) can coat a cutlet, add heft to meatballs, or transform into a crunchy toasted topping for pasta or fish fillets. Regular dried breadcrumbs are also useful.

DRIED HERBS AND SPICES

Everyone's spice cabinet looks a little different since it reflects the type of food we like to cook the most. My spice collection is both eclectic and overflowing. But you can make delicious meals with a relatively limited number of spices, including:

- Ground cumin
- Ground coriander
- Ground cinnamon
- Ground ginger
- Ground turmeric
- Ground sumac
- Smoked paprika
- Crushed red pepper
- Black peppercorns
- Dried oregano—the only dried herb I use with any regularity
- Garlic powder
- Onion powder

And, while I used to be a purist about mixing my own spice rubs and blends, I have discovered the joys of buying them and make good use of:

- Ras el hanout—a North African spice blend
- Za'atar—a blend of spices and sesame seeds used frequently in Middle Eastern cooking
- Curry powder—yes, this is a blend!
- Garam masala
- Chili powder—another blend! (not to be confused with pure ground chiles such as cayenne pepper or chipotle chile powder)
- Fajita spice blend
- Italian herb blend

And ignore any knee-jerk impulse to discard jarred spices after a certain period (six months is the advice I usually see). Instead, shake the bottle and give it a sniff. If the spice still smells vibrant, hold on to it. If there's only a faint aroma, or none at all, toss it. There's no point in taking the time to measure a spice if it won't add flavor to your dish.

Salt

There are a few kitchen essentials I make sure I am never without—peanut butter, paper towels, and olive oil to start. But absolutely number one on the list is salt. Now, unless you're making potato chips or French fries, salt isn't necessarily meant to make your food taste, well, *salty*. Rather, salt balances acidic and bitter foods and adds complexity to sweet foods. It makes everything—in a word—pop.

And I want pop in everything I eat! If I bite into a piece of pasta or broccoli or chicken, and it's just okay, the first thing I do is add a few flakes of sea salt. Nine times out of ten that does the trick and the food tastes more delicious.

There are two equally important ways to use salt. First is as you're actually cooking: salting pasta water, seasoning veggies before sliding them into the oven to roast, sprinkling it on chicken or meat before searing. And then there's finishing—think of this almost as a garnish, just as you would grind a little pepper over a finished dish. Crush a pinch of flaky sea salt in your fingers and shower it over your food. For optimally delicious food, be sure to use salt in both these ways in your cooking process. It really is a bare minimum way to add flavor.

For cooking, I use kosher salt. It's what I learned in culinary school, and I've never looked back. Kosher has a coarser grind than table salt and a cleaner flavor. I use Diamond Crystal brand; it's inexpensive and widely available, and it comes in a big enough box to make me feel secure for a while. Know that kosher salt has less sodium than table salt by volume, and that I tested these recipes with Diamond Crystal kosher. If you're using table salt, or even a different brand of kosher (such as Morton's), you may need to adjust the salt amount in each recipe. Taste often when you're cooking and add salt a little at a time. You can always add more, but it's tricky to remove it!

For finishing, look for a flaky sea salt. There are many excellent varieties available. I love Maldon, a widely available salt from England. It's sturdy enough to add some crunch to a dish, yet soft enough to crumble with my fingers.

Condiments

Condiments are like magic in a jar or bottle—they can give an instant hit of big flavor to virtually anything. Many condiments are either bursting with umami (that savory richness that makes a food irresistible) or spicy heat—or both. Many of the recipes in this book rely on a dollop or splash of this magic to really bring them to life. You can read more about my favorites in the Ingredient All-Stars section on page 16, but these are my must-haves:

- Mayonnaise
- Dijon mustard
- Ketchup
- Soy sauce or tamari
- Maple syrup
- Hot honey (the original is Mike's brand)

- Hot sauce (Cholula is my favorite)
- Harissa
- Sriracha
- Sambal oelek
- Chili crisp

THE BARE MINIMUM FREEZER

The freezer is one of the most underrated appliances in the kitchen. It's key for preventing food waste, since you can freeze leftovers for future meals. It also helps extend the life of foods like sliced bread, fresh berries, pancakes, and baked goods, which can be frozen for months. And, when it comes to bare minimum dinners, the freezer means you can have ingredients at your fingertips without worrying that they'll go bad.

The deep freeze is especially useful for keeping protein on hand. Stash ground beef, chicken, seafood fillets, and shrimp in the freezer to save yourself a trip to the supermarket. Defrost meat, chicken, and fish fillets in the refrigerator overnight. Shrimp will thaw in less than a half hour in a bowl of cold water; change the water every 10 minutes. I always buy frozen shrimp now, ever since I learned that most of the shrimp at the fish counter has already been frozen and then defrosted, shortening its shelf life in my fridge.

Most of the time I eat fresh vegetables, but there are a few that I regularly pull out of the freezer. Spinach is one, since you have to wash a boatload of fresh spinach to end up with the same amount you get in a 10-ounce package of frozen. I also like the texture of frozen peas and frozen corn. Frozen artichokes come in handy, and I've been experimenting with frozen cauliflower rice. And, while I generally prefer the texture of fresh broccoli and cauliflower, frozen works just fine in soups and stews.

I also stock a variety of frozen fruits for smoothies and other breakfast and dessert recipes, and I store chocolate chips and shredded unsweetened coconut in the freezer.

Easy Swaps

Canned chickpeas → canned cannellini beans

Kale → Swiss chard → spinach (just remember that kale needs the longest to cook)

Ground beef → ground lamb → ground turkey

Sour cream → plain whole-milk Greek yogurt → crème fraîche

Maple syrup → honey

Panko → dried breadcrumbs

INGREDIENT ALL-STARS

There are a few ingredients you'll see over and over in this book. They're the powerhouses that turn a more streamlined meal into a flavor bomb and/or the ingredients that are so versatile I reach for them a *lot*. These are the first-stringers in my house; you may find others in yours.

Flaky sea salt See my ode to Maldon on page 14.

Grated Parmesan cheese I call for the generic "Parmesan" cheese in this cookbook. But, if your budget allows, spring for authentic Parmigiano-Reggiano, made in only five provinces in Italy and aged for at least 12 months. Its flavor is unmatched—you get a satisfying blast of umami in every bite. You can buy pre-grated or a block. I usually keep both on hand, the block for grating onto pasta with a Microplane, and pre-grated for when I need a large amount of it or am in a hurry.

Every other cheese Cheese is a shortcut for richness, savoriness, saltiness, and kid-friendliness, especially in meatless meals.

Tomato paste Like Parmesan cheese, this is another ingredient that's packed with umami. Get the most bang for your buck by sautéing tomato paste in a little oil, so it caramelizes slightly. Tomato paste adds a rich depth of flavor to soups, stews, and meaty sautés with ground beef or lamb.

Hot sauce As you will see in the following recipes, my family likes a little (or a lot of) zing in our dinners, so many of the recipes call for optional hot sauce for serving. I reach for Cholula for anything vaguely Latin American, and sriracha or, more often, super-spicy sambal oelek (an Indonesian chili paste) for East Asian food. A little goes a long way!

Crushed red pepper This is how I add heat to Italian-style recipes. For maximum flavor, I sauté the flakes briefly in a little olive oil, often with garlic, before pouring the spiced oil onto cooked vegetables or pasta. But, more often, I just put the spice jar on the table for everyone to add it directly to pasta, pizza, vegetables, or soups.

Olive oil A drizzle of extra virgin olive oil on top of vegetables, soup, or pasta is a chef trick that everyone should be using at home and a super-simple way to add richness to so many meals. Of course, be sure to use an olive oil you like the taste of.

Cabbage What can't a cabbage do? I use it to add crunch to tacos, bulk to stir-fries, and veggie power to a meaty meal. It fries up beautifully into little pancakes and becomes meltingly tender when sautéed in butter. Its flavor is so mild it translates well to nearly any type of dish. It's dirt cheap, and a whole head of cabbage will keep in your fridge for up to 3 weeks and yield a *lot* of shredded or wedged cabbage. I usually buy plain old green or purple cabbage. Frilly napa has a lovely freshness but doesn't last as long—I think of it more as a sturdy lettuce. I can barely bring myself to cut into a bumpy savoy because it's so beautiful. (Somehow I manage in the end.) Bags of pre-shredded cabbage are fine, too, but plan to use within a few days of buying, as pre-chopped and shredded veggies never last as long as whole.

Scallions My favorite thing about scallions is that they're easy to prep! I use them to add a mild bite to eggs, rice, or other grains. And I often call on the greens as a garnish, instead of leafy herbs, because they're easier to clean than herbs.

Cherry tomatoes The tastiest out-of-season, supermarket tomatoes, these little guys add color and bright flavor to any dish.

Plain whole-milk Greek yogurt Creamy yogurt is the rare ingredient that adds both richness (fat) and tanginess (acid) to a dish. I use it liberally in dips and marinades and as a dollop to finish tacos or meaty recipes. It's a super-easy way to add an extra dimension of flavor and texture to so many dishes. Dial it back to reduced-fat if you must, but please, please avoid fat-free. Its texture is grainy and won't give you the same satisfying creaminess as whole-milk yogurt. My favorite brands are Wallaby and Maple Hill. And, it doesn't have to be "Greek," as long as it's extra thick. Plain whole-milk skyr (Icelandic yogurt, such as Siggi's) or another strained variety will also do the trick.

A drizzle of olive oil, sprinkle of flaky sea salt, and pinch of crushed red pepper make even the simplest dish sing.

MEAL PLANNING

In my experience, having at least a vague notion of what I'm going to cook for dinner in the coming days drastically increases the likelihood of actually doing that cooking, instead of coming home and succumbing to the siren song of ordering delivery. Some people are deeply committed meal planners, scheduling out dinners over the course of a month right down to the side dish. I admire that approach (and am a little jealous of it), but I've learned that the only right way to meal plan is the way that works for you. Whatever the specifics of your method, there are three universal steps:

1. **Have options.** This might be as simple as a list tacked up on the fridge of meals that the whole family likes. Or maybe it's a Pinterest board of dishes you enjoy or want to try. Or perhaps you have a physical file of printouts and recipes ripped from magazines. Or recipes you want to try in cookbooks, of course!

2. **Write it down.** Decide what you want to eat for the next week and write it down. Somewhere. Anywhere. It could be a dedicated Google sheet (my method), a note on your phone, or a meal planning notebook. Just don't keep the plan in your head. Trust me.

3. **Make a grocery list.** Once you have your meal plan for the week, write down all of the ingredients you need for the recipes. Check what you already have and cross those off the list. Then shop and cook!

There are two other meal planning methods I know work for some folks. One of my favorites is to assign a theme to each night—think Meatless Monday, Taco Tuesday, Italian Wednesday, etc. Even that rough structure can be useful when you're deciding what to cook. Or, simply make a plan for two to three weeks of dinners and put it on repeat. You can even keep a master grocery list.

Meal planning isn't for everyone. But if you can create even the most basic plan for the coming week, I guarantee that dinnertime will feel like less of a burden.

REDUCING FOOD WASTE

Cutting back on food waste—and food packaging—has become a key component of my cooking and eating routine and probably yours, too. And rightfully so: Reducing food waste is good for the environment (food makes up about 20 percent of our municipal solid waste) and good for your bank account (the average American family throws away about $1200 worth of food a year). Here are five things to keep in mind if you're trying to reduce food waste:

Stick to your plan. There is a reason this section comes right after the meal planning section, because the former helps prevent the latter. If you plan meals, shop for them, and then cook them, you're much less likely to have food going bad in the fridge than if you just buy random ingredients, use a few, don't know exactly what to do with the others, and end up going out or ordering in.

If you don't bring it home, it won't end up in the trash. Or, in other words, don't go overboard at the grocery store! When you shop, try to be realistic about how much you'll actually eat in a week, and just because something's on sale doesn't mean it's a good buy, especially if it's perishable and you're going to end up tossing some of it.

Eat dinner for lunch. Give supper new life as lunch the next day. Whether you're at home and heat it up in the microwave or pack it in a thermos for your kid's lunch at school or your own desk lunch, get in the habit of eating left-overs the next day. Bonus: You'll save time on lunch packing. Give your leftovers a little spark by employing your new flavor-boosting routine: a drizzle of olive oil, sprinkle of sea salt, and shower of crushed red pepper or dash of hot sauce.

Use your freezer. When you notice that produce is on its way out, pop it in the freezer to extend its life. Freeze berries in a single layer on a parchment-lined baking sheet to keep them from clumping, then transfer them to a freezer bag or other storage container once frozen. Blend herbs with olive oil in the food processor to make a basic pesto, and then freeze in ice cube trays. Most veggies benefit from being blanched (quickly cooked in boiling water) before freezing. Cook, dry, and store.

Add on. Certain dishes like frittatas, stir-fries, and soups are generally welcoming to the odds and ends of your crisper and cheese drawers. Don't be afraid to improvise a little by adding different or additional ingredients.

9 Commandments of
BARE MINIMUM DINNERS

1 **Let go of ambition (at least some of the time).**

Weeknight dinners do not need to be elaborate, Instagram-worthy, or restaurant-caliber. Good enough is great. You aren't cooking for the queen here.

2 **Lean on those Ingredient All-Stars.**

Especially when you're making a meal with a limited number of ingredients, each one has to count. There are certain ingredients (see page 16) that do more than pull their weight, often the ones packed with umami. Use them liberally.

3 **Then lean harder.**

In the same vein, think about what's making you really want to eat this food and consider adding just a little more. A good dish is all about the balance between sweet, salty, savory, tangy, and spicy. But sometimes putting your finger on the scale and adding a little more of whatever that especially delicious ingredient is—maybe a sprinkle more Parm or a touch more butter or a few extra olives—can make a meal more deeply pleasurable.

4 **Season to taste.**

Just because you've followed a recipe to the letter doesn't mean it will taste delicious to you. The best strategy is to taste the food before serving it to see if it needs a little more seasoning, aka salt, pepper, or a spritz of lemon or lime.

5 **Shop smart.**

Run-of-the-mill grocery stores have come a long way. Take advantage of the excellent dinnertime shortcuts available now, especially premade Indian simmer sauces, marinara, enchilada sauce, and salsa. They can make a meal.

It's about more than the food.

Whether we live with partners, kids, or on our own, dinnertime is usually one of the set points of our day. While there's something decadent and delicious about eating in front of the television or screen sometimes, on most nights try to make the meal a moment to sit at a table, take a deep breath, enjoy what you're eating, and maybe even talk to each other (or yourself!).

Be flexible.

Don't let the fact that you don't have a specific herb or spice or other ingredient deter you from a recipe. Think about (or Google!) what a good substitute would be and use that. Or, if it isn't a main ingredient in the recipe, just leave it out. It will be fine, and if it's not you'll know for next time.

Use every minute of prep time.

If a sheet-pan dinner is roasting for 15 minutes or even if a pasta sauce is just simmering for 5, use the time to get a head start on cleanup. Empty the dish rack or dishwasher. Wash any measuring cups and spoons you used. Put away jars of ingredients. Or, if you're squared away on the cleanup front, set the table, fill glasses, and put out condiments.

Enjoy the process—or don't!

Some nights I put on a podcast, pour a small glass of wine, and glide through dinner prep. Other nights I'm frazzled and on edge, and want to just eat already. Both of these emotional states are equally valid. Cooking isn't always a joy and it isn't always a headache. Make peace with whatever mood you're in and just keep going. The meal will get done either way, and hopefully it's satisfying enough to make it all worthwhile.

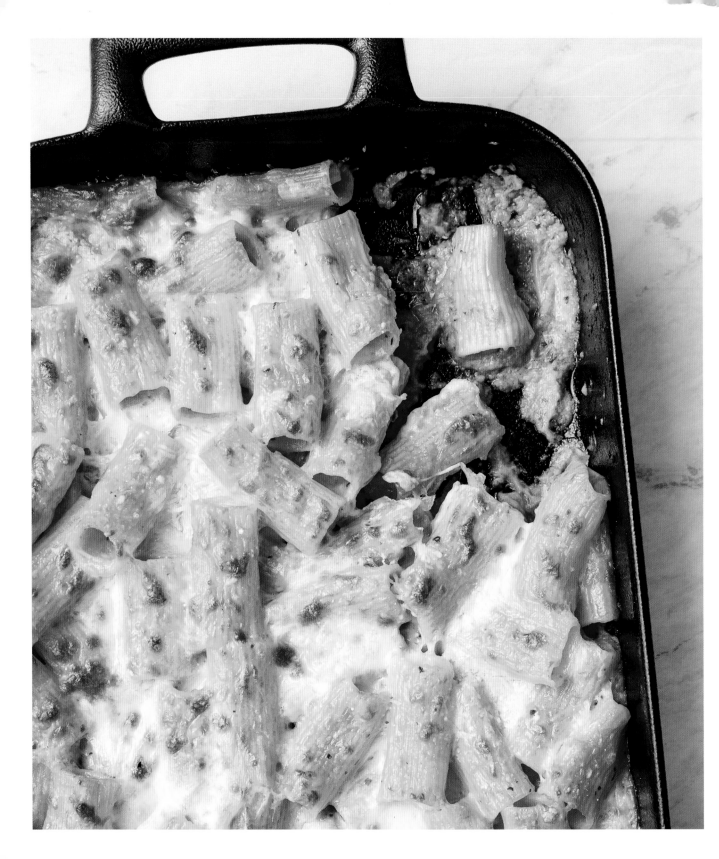

MY NONNEGOTIABLE DINNER RULES

1. **There must be a vegetable.** Maybe it's my years writing for families with young kids or my stint working at *Health* magazine, but to me, dinner just isn't dinner without some vegetable involved. About half the time at my house that means a quickie green salad. It fulfills the vegetable requirement in about 60 seconds flat! (See page 193 for my Any Green Leaf Salad recipe.)

2. **There must be enough food to satiate you.** We've all had those dinners that are good but leave you feeling peckish a half hour later. Dinner should fill you up, even if you have to add on at the last minute. Whenever my family and I find ourselves not quite satisfied at the end of a meal, we bring out some cheese on a cutting board. That usually does the trick.

3. **There must be at least one part of the meal that you're really looking forward to eating.** I want to *enjoy* my dinner. It has taken me years, but I finally realized that unless there's something on the menu that I am actively anticipating, I'm much more likely to throw in the towel on cooking and order something that I'm craving instead. That special something might be spicy-sweet roasted brussels sprouts, a rice bowl with punchy kimchi, or a golden breaded chicken cutlet. It doesn't have to be a whole dish but rather any element of a dish that's big on flavor and satisfaction.

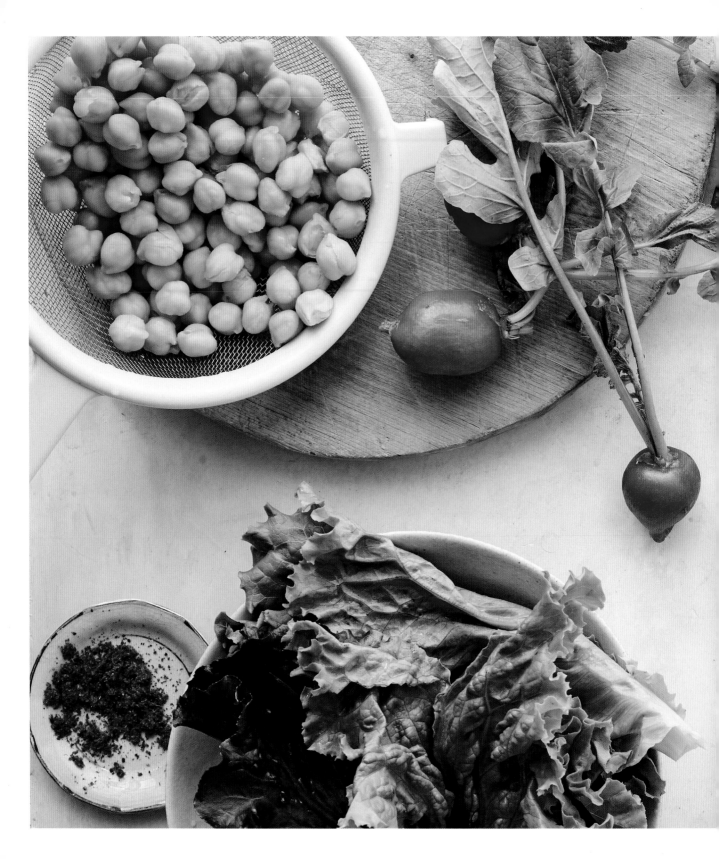

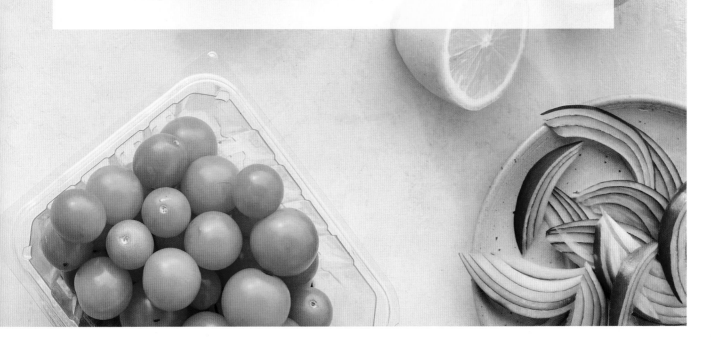

BARE MINIMUM
Time

Recipes Ready in 30 Minutes or Less

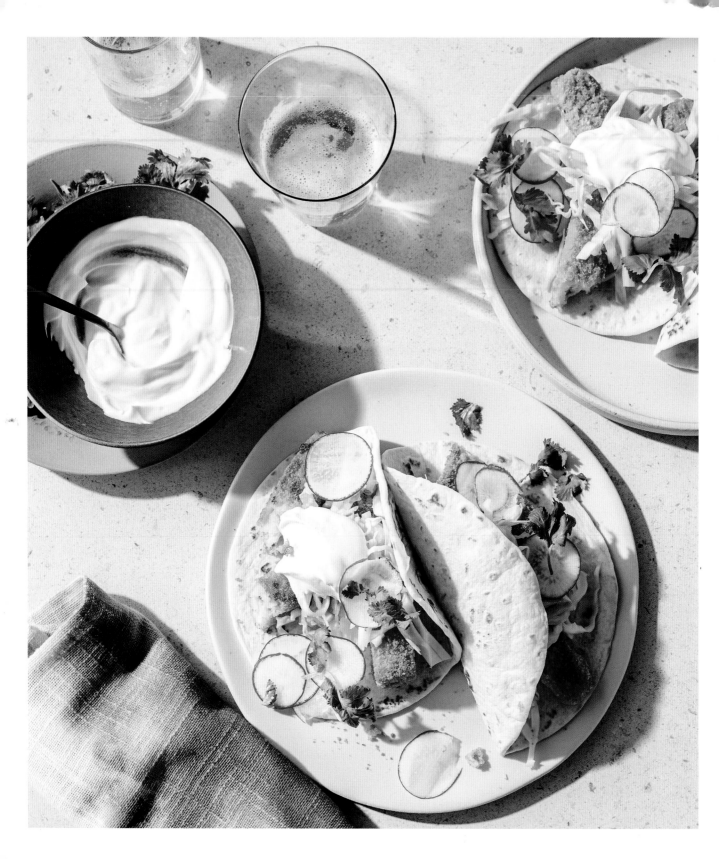

Fish Stick Tacos

MAKES 4 SERVINGS

This is the original bare minimum dinner in my household—and one of two dinners my husband feels utterly confident making. Sure, I've grilled or even deep-fried fish for tacos, but frozen fish sticks are a genius alternative. To quickly warm the tortillas, wrap them in a damp kitchen towel, put the bundle on a plate, and microwave on high for 60 to 90 seconds. Don't like (or don't have) sauerkraut? Skip it and add another tablespoon of vinegar to the cabbage.

16 frozen fish sticks (about 1 pound)

4 cups shredded cabbage (about 12 ounces)

1 cup refrigerated sauerkraut

1 tablespoon apple cider vinegar

¾ teaspoon kosher salt

8 small flour or corn tortillas, warmed

DRESS IT UP Sour cream or plain Greek yogurt, hot sauce, chopped radishes, cilantro sprigs

Ingredient Tip

Look for sauerkraut in your supermarket's refrigerated section and check to be sure the label says "raw," "live," or "fermented." This ensures that you'll be getting gut-friendly probiotics in every bite, plus a fresher flavor than what you'd find in shelf-stable jars.

1. Bake the fish sticks according to the package directions.

2. While the fish sticks are cooking, combine the cabbage, sauerkraut, vinegar, and salt in a medium bowl. Toss well and let sit until ready to serve, tossing occasionally.

3. Place two fish sticks on each tortilla and top with some of the cabbage mixture. Add sour cream, hot sauce, radishes, and/or cilantro, if desired. Serve the remaining cabbage mixture on the side as a salad.

Provini Pasta

MAKES 4 SERVINGS

There is a small Italian restaurant called Provini in our neighborhood in Brooklyn where we are regulars. This dish is a riff on one of our very favorite orders there. I adore broccoli rabe, a deliciously bitter green that's part of the turnip family, but you could substitute broccoli florets. If you don't have toasted walnuts on hand, toast them while the pasta water is coming to a boil.

Kosher salt, for the pasta water

1 pound orecchiette

1 bunch broccoli rabe, woody ends removed, cut into 2-inch pieces

2 tablespoons olive oil, plus more for drizzling

½ cup chopped walnuts, toasted (see page 11)

Grated zest of 1 lemon

DRESS IT UP Flaky sea salt

1. Bring a large pot of well-salted water to a boil. Add the orecchiette and cook for 5 minutes. Stir in the broccoli rabe and continue to cook until the pasta is al dente, 4 to 5 more minutes, stirring occasionally. Reserve 1 cup cooking water and drain. Return the pasta and broccoli rabe to the pot.

2. Add the olive oil and half of the reserved cooking water to the pot. Stir vigorously to break up the broccoli rabe, adding more pasta water if a looser consistency is desired. Serve topped with the walnuts and lemon zest. Drizzle with more olive oil and season with flaky sea salt, if desired.

Cooking Tip

Be sure to generously salt the cooking water for pasta and quick-cooking vegetables. The water should taste well seasoned, almost like the sea.

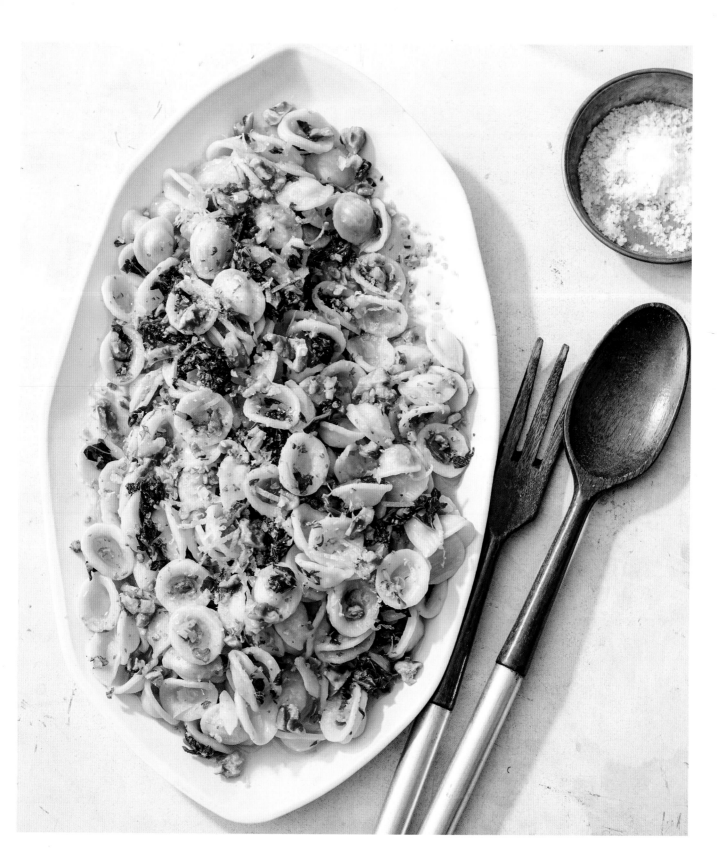

Ginger-Scallion Turkey Burgers

MAKES 4 SERVINGS

These burgers have it all: a hit of flavor from the ginger, crunch from the lettuce, and creaminess from the avocado. Use a cast-iron pan if you have one—it helps make for even browning on both sides of the patty.

1 pound 93% lean ground turkey

2 scallions, trimmed and chopped

2 teaspoons grated fresh ginger

1 teaspoon kosher salt

1 tablespoon canola or other neutral oil

4 burger buns (preferably brioche), toasted

4 leaves butter lettuce

1 avocado, pitted, peeled, and sliced

DRESS IT UP Mayonnaise mixed with sriracha

1. In a large bowl, combine the ground turkey, scallions, ginger, and salt and mix well with a fork.

2. Heat the oil in a large skillet over medium-high heat. Form the turkey mixture into 4 patties and add to the pan. Cook until browned and cooked through (165°F on an instant-read thermometer), 4 to 5 minutes per side. Reduce the heat to medium if the burgers are browning too quickly.

3. Serve the burgers on the toasted buns with lettuce and avocado slices, plus mayo and sriracha, if desired.

ROUND IT OUT Everyday Broccoli (page 197), Quick Cukes (page 218), or Spicy-Sweet Roasted Brussels Sprouts (page 206)

Cooking Tip

When forming the patties, use your thumb to make an indentation in the top side. This helps the patties cook evenly, and you'll avoid the dreaded domed burger.

Tortellini en Brodo

MAKES 4 SERVINGS

This Italian classic is traditionally made with homemade chicken broth. For a speedy yet satisfying weeknight dinner, use boxed broth livened up with lemon.

4 cups chicken broth (32 ounces)

Juice of ½ lemon (about 1 tablespoon)

1 12–13-ounce package refrigerated or frozen tortellini

½ teaspoon kosher salt

1 bunch Swiss chard, stems removed and leaves roughly chopped

Olive oil, for drizzling

Freshly ground black pepper to taste

DRESS IT UP Crushed red pepper, grated Parmesan cheese

1. In a large pot, bring the chicken broth and 2 cups water to a boil. Stir in the lemon juice and tortellini. Cook until the tortellini is just tender, 2 to 3 minutes for most refrigerated varieties. Remove from the heat.

2. Stir in the salt and chard. Cover and let sit until the chard is wilted, about 2 minutes.

3. Ladle into bowls and top with a drizzle of olive oil and a few grinds of black pepper. Pass the crushed red pepper and Parm at the table, if desired.

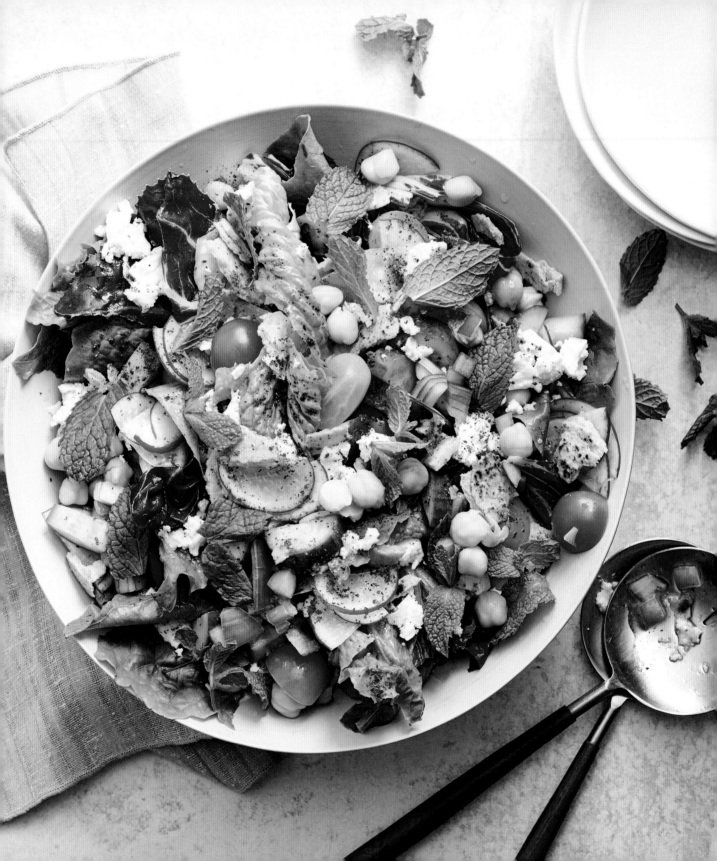

Lemony Chopped Salad with Pita

MAKES 4 SERVINGS

This bright, fresh, crunchy dinner is a riff on fattoush, a Lebanese salad made with torn and toasted pita. I've bulked it up with chickpeas and feta to give it more staying power.

1 15-ounce can chickpeas, rinsed and drained

¼ cup chopped red onion

2 tablespoons red wine vinegar

1¼ teaspoons kosher salt, divided

2 pita bread rounds

Juice of 1 lemon (about 2 tablespoons)

1 teaspoon honey

½ cup olive oil

4 mini (Persian) cucumbers, trimmed

2 radishes, trimmed

1 pint cherry tomatoes

8 cups loosely packed salad greens (about 4 ounces)

4 ounces feta cheese

DRESS IT UP Torn mint leaves, ground sumac

1. Preheat the oven to 350°F.

2. While the oven is preheating, put the chickpeas and onion in a large bowl. Add the red wine vinegar and ¼ teaspoon of the salt. Toss to combine and set aside.

3. Tear the pita into bite-sized pieces and place on a rimmed baking sheet. Bake for 10 minutes. Let cool on the baking sheet.

4. While the pita is baking, make the dressing: Whisk together the lemon juice, honey, and another ¾ teaspoon salt in a small bowl. Whisk in the olive oil.

5. Prepare the vegetables: Slice the cucumbers into chunky half-moons and the radishes into thin half-moons. Cut the tomatoes in half. Add the veggies to the bowl with the chickpeas and toss to combine. Add the pita and pour over the dressing. Add the salad greens and remaining ¼ teaspoon salt and toss to coat. Crumble the feta into the bowl and gently toss to combine. Serve topped with torn mint leaves and/or a sprinkle of sumac, if desired.

BARE MINIMUM *Time*

Tuna and White Bean Salad

MAKES 3 SERVINGS

I have been making variations of this salad for years. I love the meatiness of the tuna, the creaminess of the beans, and the pop of flavor from the olives or capers. This version includes cucumber, which adds a pleasing snap to every bite. Serve as is, on toast, or over salad greens.

1 15-ounce can cannellini beans, rinsed, drained, and patted dry

3 tablespoons olive oil

½ teaspoon kosher salt

Juice of ½ lemon (about 1 tablespoon), plus more if needed

1 6–7-ounce jar tuna in olive oil, drained

2 mini (Persian) cucumbers, trimmed and chopped (about 1 cup)

¼ cup pitted olives, roughly chopped, or 2 tablespoons capers

Put the beans in a large bowl. Using a fork, coarsely mash about half of them. Add the olive oil, salt, and the lemon juice. Stir to combine. Add the tuna, cucumber, and olives. Taste, and add more lemon or salt, if desired.

ROUND IT OUT Toast and/or Any Green Leaf Salad (page 193)

Caesar-ish Kale Salad

MAKES 4 SERVINGS

This veggie-full—yet totally satisfying—dinner will come together even faster if you already have hard-boiled eggs on hand.

4 large eggs

¼ cup mayonnaise

3 tablespoons olive oil

1 tablespoon Dijon mustard

Juice of ½ lemon (about 1 tablespoon)

½ teaspoon Worcestershire sauce

½ teaspoon kosher salt, divided

Freshly ground black pepper to taste

1 bunch curly kale, stems removed and leaves chopped (about 10 cups)

¼ cup grated Parmesan cheese (about 1 ounce)

½ cup chopped toasted walnuts or almonds

Cooking Tip

I have tried many ways of hard-boiling eggs over the years, including steaming them and cooking them in the Instant Pot. All these methods have their perks, but I find myself returning to stove-top boiling (see step 1) again and again. A couple more hard-boiled egg tips: If you're not eating the eggs right away, store them in the fridge in their shells. And, the best way to get hard-cooked eggs to peel easily? Start with eggs that have been in your fridge for at least a week. Egg whites shrink slightly as they age, resulting in more space between the egg and the shell, which makes it easier to peel.

1. Bring a medium pot of water to a boil. Carefully lower the eggs into the water, reduce the heat to a simmer, and cook for 11 minutes. Using a slotted spoon, transfer the eggs to a bowl of ice-cold water.

2. While the eggs are cooking, whisk together the mayonnaise, olive oil, mustard, lemon juice, Worcestershire sauce, ¼ teaspoon of the salt, and lots of pepper in a large bowl. Add the kale, and, using tongs, toss well until all the leaves are coated. Add the Parmesan cheese and toss again.

3. Divide the kale into 4 shallow bowls. Peel and slice the eggs, adding one to each bowl. Sprinkle with the remaining ¼ teaspoon salt and more pepper. Top with the nuts and serve.

V MAKE IT MEATLESS Skip the Worcestershire sauce and add a pinch more salt.

Spicy Sloppy Joes

MAKES 4 SERVINGS

I don't really like traditional Sloppy Joes. They're just too darn sweet for my palate. But I love the idea *of Sloppy Joes, the burger's more casual, slightly messy cousin. This Korean-flavored version has made a convert out of me. It's deeply savory with just a touch of sweet and a hit of spice. If you can't find gochujang, an increasingly easy-to-locate Korean chili paste, substitute sriracha. Both condiments pack a punch, so use just 1 tablespoon in this recipe if you prefer less heat.*

1 teaspoon toasted sesame oil

1 pound lean ground beef

2 cloves garlic, sliced

½ cup tomato puree

3 tablespoons soy sauce or tamari

1–2 tablespoons gochujang (Korean chili paste)

1 tablespoon brown sugar

Juice of ½ lime

4 burger buns (preferably brioche), toasted

DRESS IT UP Sliced scallions

1. Heat the sesame oil in a large skillet over medium-high heat. Add the ground beef and garlic. Cook, breaking up the beef with a wooden spoon, until no longer pink, about 5 minutes. Transfer to a colander to drain the fat, then return the beef to the pan.

2. While the beef browns, stir together the tomato puree, ¼ cup water, soy sauce, gochujang, and brown sugar in a medium bowl.

3. Pour the tomato mixture over the beef and stir to combine. Bring the mixture to a simmer and cook, partially covered, over medium-low heat for about 10 minutes. Stir in the lime juice and scallions, if using. Serve the beef mixture on the toasted buns.

ROUND IT OUT Quick Cukes (page 218), Savory Fruit Salad (page 217), or Roasted Shredded Brussels Sprouts (page 205)

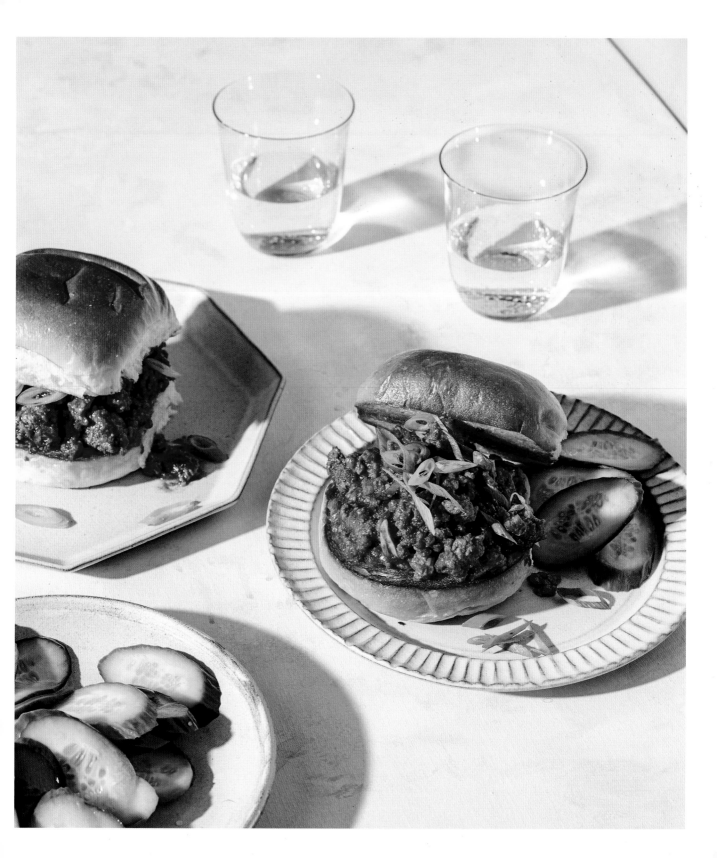

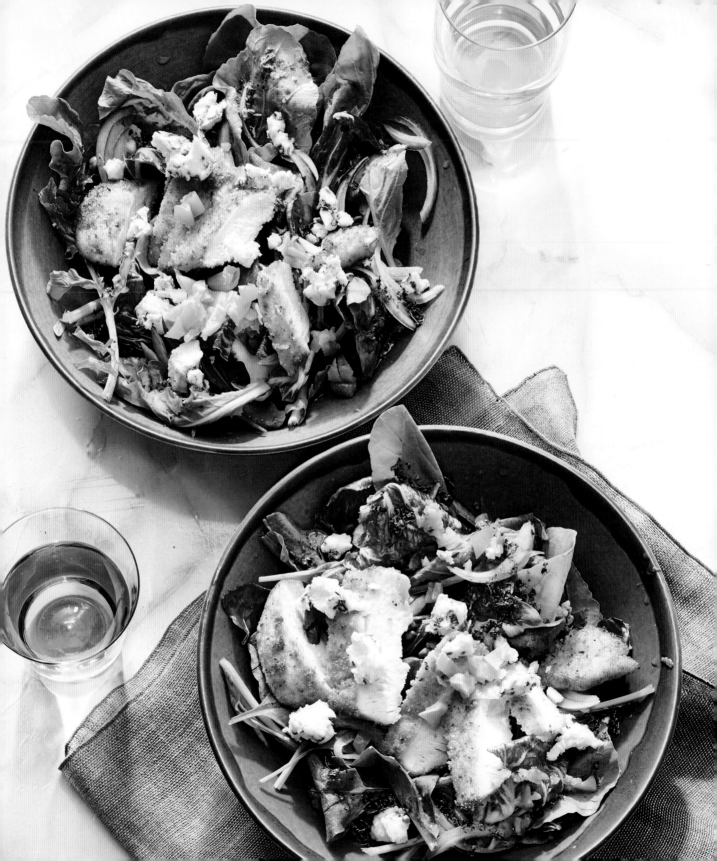

Crispy Chicken Salad

MAKES 4 SERVINGS

This is exactly the type of salad that I crave: one with lots of delicious, savory, salty things that make eating a bowl of greens a pleasure.

1 pound thin chicken breast cutlets

1 teaspoon kosher salt, divided

½ cup dried breadcrumbs

1½ teaspoons Italian seasoning, divided

¼ cup plus 3 tablespoons olive oil, divided, plus more if needed

10 cups loosely packed salad greens (such as a combination of red leaf lettuce, arugula, and radicchio; 5–7 ounces)

¼ cup thinly sliced red onion

2 tablespoons capers

1 tablespoon red wine vinegar

2 ounces semi-firm salty cheese (such as blue or feta), cubed or crumbled

DRESS IT UP 3 or 4 jarred pepperoncini, finely chopped

1. Sprinkle the chicken cutlets on both sides with ½ teaspoon of the salt. Combine the breadcrumbs and ½ teaspoon of the Italian seasoning on a plate. Press the seasoned cutlets into the breadcrumbs to coat.

2. Heat ¼ cup of the olive oil in a large skillet over medium-high heat. Cooking in batches if necessary, sauté the cutlets until golden brown and cooked through, 3 to 4 minutes per side. (Add more oil for a second batch, or if the pan seems dry.) Transfer to a paper towel–lined plate.

3. Combine the salad greens, red onion, and capers in a large bowl. Add the remaining 3 tablespoons olive oil, red wine vinegar, remaining 1 teaspoon Italian seasoning, and remaining ½ teaspoon salt. Toss with tongs, then divide among 4 shallow bowls. Slice the chicken and divide among the salads. Top with the cheese and pepperoncini, if using.

∨ MAKE IT MEATLESS Skip the chicken and top each salad with 1 sliced hard-boiled egg.

Good Money Flounder

I'd been calling this Flounder Piccata, since it's a remake of the classic Italian chicken dish. But one time I made it, my husband said (between bites), "I would pay good money for this in a restaurant." And the new name has stuck. Use any thin, white fish here, such as lemon sole or tilapia.

4 6-ounce flounder fillets

¾ teaspoon kosher salt, plus a pinch more

½ cup all-purpose flour

2 tablespoons olive oil, plus more if needed

¼ cup white wine

1 tablespoon fresh lemon juice

1 tablespoon capers

1½ tablespoons unsalted butter

1. Season the flounder on both sides with the salt. Put the flour in a shallow dish and press the seasoned fish into the flour, shaking off any excess.

2. Heat the olive oil in a large nonstick or cast-iron skillet over medium-high heat. Add 2 of the fillets and sauté until golden on the bottom, about 3 minutes. Carefully flip the fillets and continue sautéing until cooked through, about 2 minutes more. Transfer to a serving platter or plates. If the pan seems dry, add another tablespoon of olive oil. Repeat with the remaining fillets, then transfer them to the platter.

3. Reduce the heat to medium-low. Add the wine to the pan and scrape up any brown bits on the bottom of the pan. Let the wine reduce by about half (this will happen in under a minute!). Stir in the lemon juice, capers, and a pinch of salt. Remove the pan from the heat. Stir in the butter until melted, then pour the sauce over the fish.

ROUND IT OUT Any Green Leaf Salad (page 193), crusty bread, or roasted potatoes

Lamb Pita Pizzas

MAKES 4 SERVINGS

Sumac, a spice popular in the Middle East, is one of those ingredients that can really transform a dish. Its bright, citrusy flavor makes meat pop, and I especially love to use it with lamb. Thankfully, sumac is more widely available now than ever, but if you can't find it (or ran out, as happens to me all too often), just grate lots of lemon zest over the pizza.

4 pita bread rounds (white or whole wheat)

1 pound ground lamb

4 cloves garlic, sliced

2 teaspoons ground sumac

1 teaspoon ground cumin

¾ teaspoon kosher salt

1 pint cherry tomatoes, halved

3 tablespoons plain whole-milk Greek yogurt, plus more for serving

DRESS IT UP Chopped cilantro, crushed red pepper

ROUND IT OUT Any Green Leaf Salad (page 193) or Peels-On Cumin-Roasted Carrots (page 201; start these first and continue roasting them on the bottom rack while the pizzas bake)

1. Preheat the oven to 400°F. Line two rimmed baking sheets with parchment paper.

2. Put the pitas on the prepared baking sheets and bake for 10 minutes; let cool slightly.

3. While the pitas bake, heat a large sauté pan over medium-high heat. Add the lamb and garlic. Cook, breaking up the lamb with a wooden spoon, until no longer pink, about 5 minutes. If there is a lot of fat in the pan, pour off most of it. Lower the heat to medium and stir in the sumac, cumin, salt, and tomatoes. Cover the pan and cook until the tomatoes have deflated, about 5 minutes. Scrape up any brown bits on the bottom of the pan.

4. Spread the yogurt evenly over the pitas. Divide the lamb mixture on top of the yogurt-topped pitas. Bake for 5 minutes. Cut each pita into quarters and serve with more yogurt, if desired, plus chopped cilantro and crushed red pepper if dressing it up.

Cacio e Pepe Mac 'n' Cheese

MAKES 4 TO 6 SERVINGS

This creamy, delicious crowd-pleaser is a great excuse to clean out the odds and ends of your cheese drawer; just be sure to choose good melters. The recipe requires grinding a full teaspoon of pepper. If you've got a pint-sized kitchen helper, I recommend enlisting them for that task.

¾ teaspoon kosher salt, plus more for the pasta water

1 pound fusilli or other short pasta

4 tablespoons (½ stick) unsalted butter

¼ cup all-purpose flour

3 cups whole milk (2% will work in a pinch)

2 cups shredded cheddar, Gruyère, or fontina cheese (or a combination; about 8 ounces)

½ cup finely grated pecorino Romano cheese (about 2 ounces)

1 teaspoon freshly ground black pepper, or more to taste

1. Bring a large pot of well-salted water to a boil. Cook the fusilli according to the package directions. Drain and return to the pot.

2. While the pasta is cooking, melt the butter in a medium pot over medium heat. Whisk in the flour and continue whisking for 2 minutes as the mixture (the roux) bubbles and turns a light golden color. Gradually add the milk, whisking all the while. Increase the heat to medium-high and bring the mixture to a simmer, whisking frequently. Simmer for 3 minutes.

3. Remove the sauce from the heat. Stir in the salt and cheeses. Pour the sauce over the drained pasta and stir to combine. Add the pepper and stir once more.

ROUND IT OUT Any Green Leaf Salad (page 193) or Everyday Broccoli (page 197)

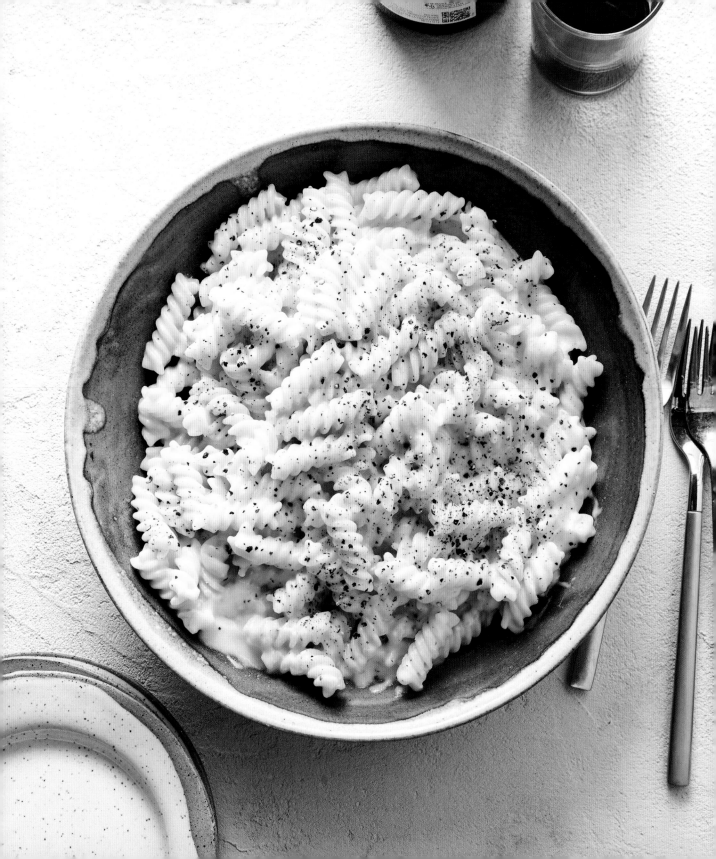

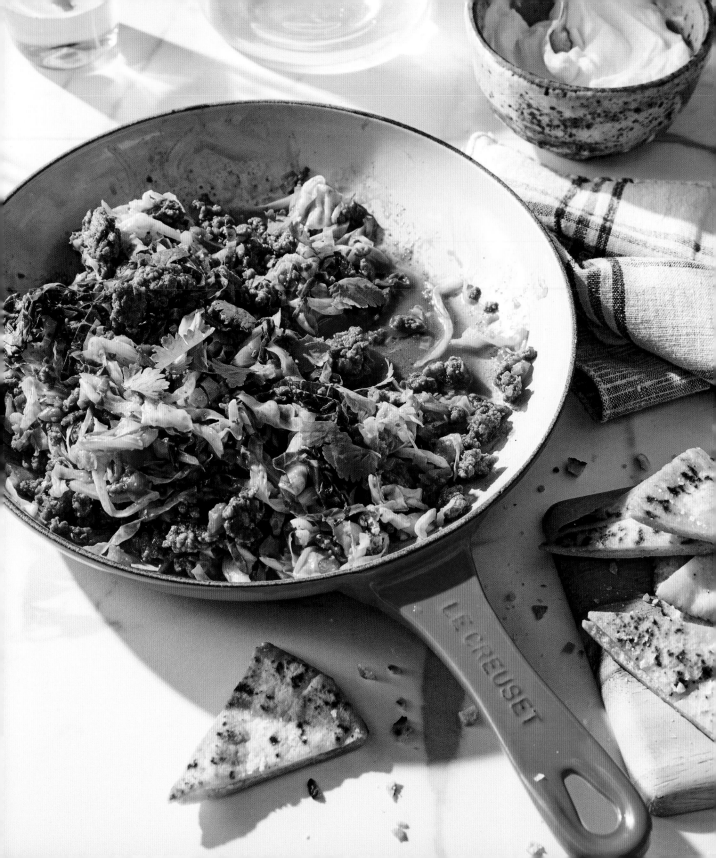

Skillet Harissa Beef and Cabbage

MAKES 3 SERVINGS

This recipe doubles easily; just be sure to use a very large skillet.

1 tablespoon olive oil

1 pound ground beef

1½ teaspoons kosher salt, divided

2 teaspoons ground cumin

4 cups shredded cabbage (about 12 ounces)

¼ cup harissa

Juice of ½ lemon (about 1 tablespoon)

Pita chips, for serving

DRESS IT UP Chopped cilantro, plain Greek yogurt or sour cream

1. Heat the olive oil in a large skillet over medium-high heat. Add the beef, 1 teaspoon of the salt, and the cumin. Cook, breaking up the beef with a wooden spoon, until no longer pink, about 5 minutes.

2. Add the cabbage and remaining ½ teaspoon salt. Cook, stirring, until the cabbage is just wilted, about 2 minutes. Remove from the heat and stir in the harissa and lemon juice. Top with cilantro and/or dollops of Greek yogurt, if desired, and serve with pita chips.

Turkey Enchilada Bowls

MAKES 4 SERVINGS

Jarred enchilada sauce is one of those shortcuts I wholeheartedly endorse. Yes, you can make your own. But for a busy weeknight, a high-quality store-bought brand (I like Frontera) is nothing to feel guilty about. You can substitute ground beef or ground chicken for the turkey.

1 cup white rice (or brown, but it will take longer)

1 pint cherry tomatoes, halved

2 tablespoons finely chopped red onion

Juice of ½ lime

¾ teaspoon salt, divided

1 tablespoon canola or other neutral oil

1 pound 93% lean ground turkey

1 cup enchilada sauce

½ cup crumbled cotija cheese or shredded cheddar (about 2 ounces)

DRESS IT UP Chopped cilantro, hot sauce

1. Cook the rice according to the package directions.

2. In the meantime, combine the tomatoes, red onion, lime juice, and ¼ teaspoon of the salt in a medium bowl. Set aside.

3. Heat the oil in a large skillet over medium-high heat. Add the turkey and remaining ½ teaspoon salt. Cook, breaking up the turkey with a spoon, until no longer pink, about 5 minutes. Add the enchilada sauce and simmer for 2 minutes.

4. Divide the rice into 4 bowls. Top with the turkey mixture, tomato mixture, and cheese. Sprinkle with cilantro and serve with hot sauce, if desired.

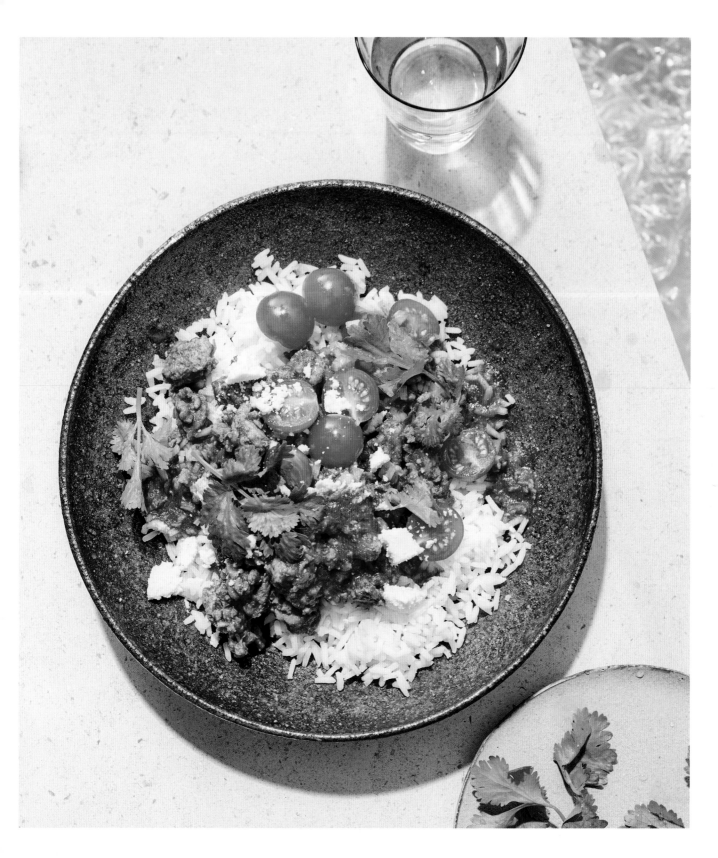

Meaty Meatless Filling

MAKES 3 TO 4 SERVINGS

Mushrooms, walnuts, and beans stand in for ground beef in this filling with Mexican flavors. Use it in tacos, burritos, or a burrito bowl with all of your favorite fixings.

2 tablespoons canola or other neutral oil

8 ounces button or cremini mushrooms, stems removed and caps finely chopped

½ cup walnuts, finely chopped

1 15-ounce can pinto beans, rinsed and drained

1 tablespoon tomato paste

2 teaspoons adobo sauce (from canned chipotle chiles in adobo sauce)

1 teaspoon ground cumin

1 teaspoon chili powder

1 teaspoon kosher salt

1. Heat the oil in a large skillet over medium-high heat. Add the mushrooms and cook, stirring occasionally, until the mushrooms are golden and most of their liquid has been cooked out, about 5 minutes. Reduce the heat to medium, add the walnuts, and cook for about 2 more minutes, stirring frequently.

2. Add the pinto beans, tomato paste, adobo sauce, cumin, chili powder, and salt. Cook, stirring, for 1 minute. Add ¼ cup water and stir to combine, gently mashing some of the beans for a thicker consistency. Simmer and cook until most of the water is absorbed, 1 to 2 more minutes. Serve immediately or store in an airtight container in the refrigerator for up to 3 days or in the freezer for up to 3 months.

Ingredient Tip

What to do with the rest of the can of chipotle chiles in adobo sauce once you've used some of it in this, or any other, recipe? Divide the chiles between cavities in an ice cube tray, and cover equally with the remaining sauce in the can. Cover and freeze until solid. Transfer the cubes to a freezer bag or other storage container and keep in the freezer for up to 6 months. Anytime you need a chipotle chile and/or some adobo sauce, place a cube or two in a small bowl, cover with a paper towel, and microwave for 30 to 60 seconds.

Sweet-and-Tangy Beef and Broccoli

MAKES 4 SERVINGS

To make thinly slicing steak easier, place the meat in the freezer for a half hour before slicing. You can replace the beef in this recipe with pork tenderloin or boneless, skinless chicken breasts. Those also slice more easily when slightly frozen.

1 cup white rice (or brown, but it will take longer)

¼ cup soy sauce or tamari

2 tablespoons maple syrup

1 tablespoon rice vinegar

1 tablespoon cornstarch

2 tablespoons toasted sesame oil, divided

8 ounces strip steak, thinly sliced

1 teaspoon kosher salt, divided

1 large bunch broccoli, cut into florets

DRESS IT UP Sriracha or sambal oelek

V MAKE IT MEATLESS Place a 14-ounce block of extra-firm tofu on a paper towel–lined plate. Top with another paper towel and another plate. Place a box of broth or can of tomatoes on the top plate to weight it down. Let the tofu drain for about 10 minutes, then cut it into cubes. Prepare the recipe as written, but omit the beef and skip step 3. Add the tofu to the pan after the sauce in step 5, and stir to warm.

1. Cook the rice according to the package directions.

2. Meanwhile, in a small bowl, stir together ½ cup water, the soy sauce, maple syrup, vinegar, and cornstarch.

3. Heat 1 tablespoon of the sesame oil in a large skillet or wok over medium-high heat. Add the steak and sprinkle with ½ teaspoon of the salt. Cook undisturbed until browned on the bottom, then stir and continue cooking until almost completely browned, 2 to 3 minutes more. Transfer the beef to a bowl and wipe out the pan if there's liquid in it.

4. Add the remaining 1 tablespoon sesame oil to the pan. Add the broccoli and remaining ½ teaspoon salt. Cook, stirring, until lightly browned, about 2 minutes. Add ½ cup water and cook until the broccoli is just tender and the water has mostly evaporated, about 3 minutes.

5. Return the beef and any accumulated juices to the pan, along with the soy sauce mixture. Cook, stirring, until the sauce is thickened, about 1 minute. Serve over the rice with sriracha or sambal oelek, if desired.

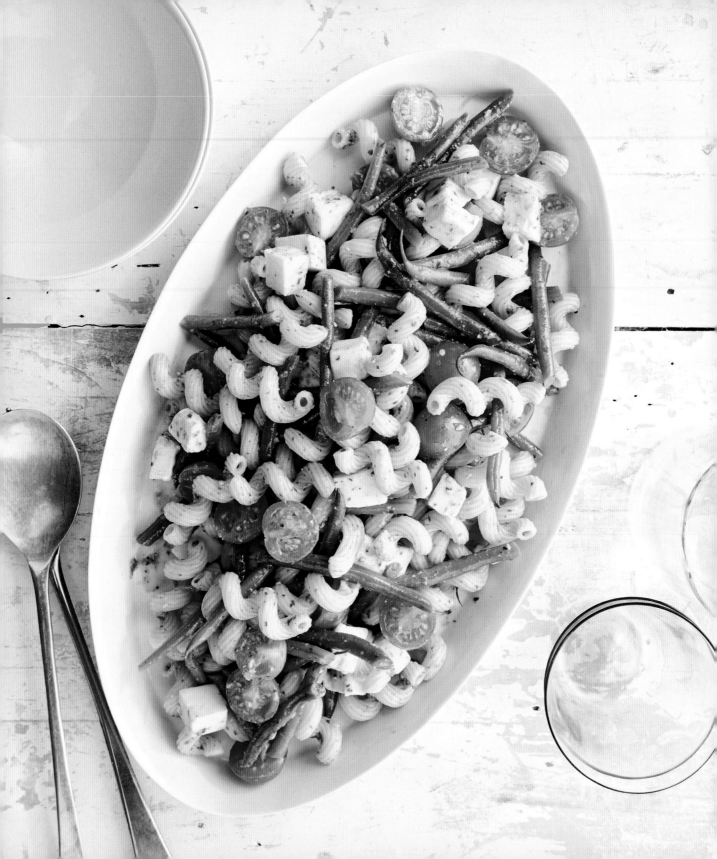

Summery Pesto Pasta

MAKES 4 SERVINGS

If you have homemade pesto, it won't find a better home than in this warm pasta salad. But store-bought can be delicious, too. For the freshest taste, look for a brand in the supermarket's refrigerated section, not jarred on the shelf.

¾ teaspoon kosher salt, plus more for the pasta water

12 ounces cherry tomatoes, halved

3 tablespoons olive oil

1 tablespoon red wine vinegar

12 ounces short spiral pasta (such as fusilli or cavatappi)

8 ounces haricots verts or green beans, trimmed and halved

⅓ cup basil pesto

8 ounces fresh mozzarella cheese, cut into small cubes

DRESS IT UP Grated Parmesan cheese

1. Bring a large pot of generously salted water to a boil.

2. While the water is coming to a boil, put the cherry tomatoes in a large bowl. Add the olive oil, red wine vinegar, and salt and stir. Let sit while you cook the pasta and haricots verts.

3. Add the pasta to the boiling water and cook according to the package directions. About 2 minutes before the pasta is finished, add the haricots verts (if using green beans, add them 3 minutes before). Drain.

4. Add the pasta and beans to the tomatoes in the bowl. Stir to coat. Let sit for 5 minutes.

5. Stir in the pesto. Add the mozzarella, toss, and serve with grated Parm, if desired.

Scallop and Asparagus Salad

MAKES 4 SERVINGS

It's unusual to combine seafood and cheese in a dish, but the Parm in this recipe adds a satisfying, savory richness that's worth breaking the rules for.

4 tablespoons olive oil, divided

1 pound sea scallops, rinsed and well dried

1¼ teaspoons kosher salt, divided

Freshly ground black pepper to taste

1 bunch asparagus, woody ends discarded and spears cut crosswise into thirds

8 cups loosely packed baby arugula (about 4 ounces)

1 lemon

Shaved Parmesan cheese, for serving

Ingredient Tip

Before cooking, use your fingers to gently remove the small rectangular muscle found on most scallops.

1. Heat 2 tablespoons of the olive oil in a large nonstick or cast-iron pan over medium-high heat. Sprinkle both sides of the scallops with ½ teaspoon of the salt and a few grinds of pepper. Add the scallops to the hot pan and cook undisturbed until they are golden and release easily from the pan, 2 to 3 minutes. (If they don't release easily, let them cook for another 30 seconds and then try again.) Gently turn them over with tongs and cook for another minute. Transfer to a plate.

2. Reduce the heat to medium and add the asparagus and another ¼ teaspoon salt to the pan. Cook for 2 minutes, stirring frequently. Add 2 tablespoons water, cover, and cook until just tender, about 2 more minutes. Remove the pan from the heat.

3. In a large bowl, toss the arugula with the remaining 2 tablespoons olive oil and remaining ½ teaspoon salt. Divide into 4 shallow bowls. Top with the scallops and asparagus. Zest the lemon over the plates, then cut the lemon in half and squeeze the juice from one half over the salads. Top with shaved Parmesan and serve.

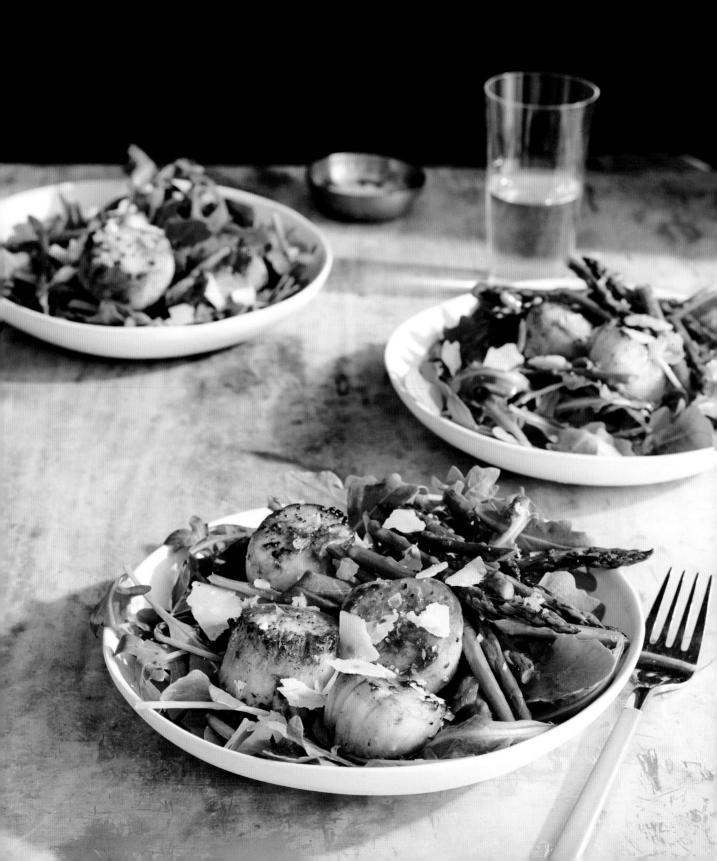

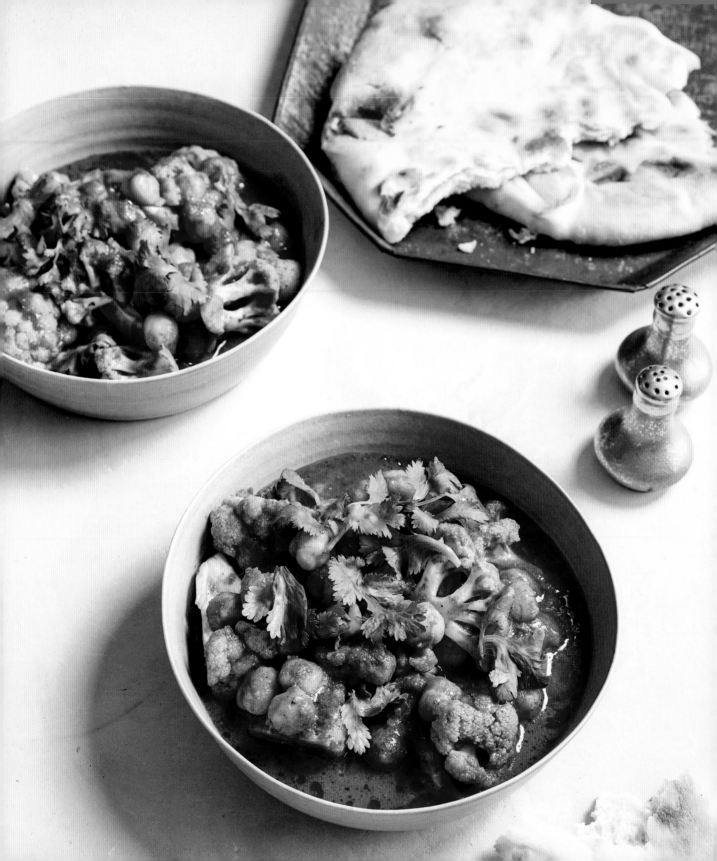

Cauliflower and Chickpea Tikka Masala

MAKES 3 TO 4 SERVINGS

This ultra-easy recipe is a great example of how a jarred sauce can make dinner a snap. Feel free to skip the rice and serve with store-bought naan or pita bread instead.

1½ cups white rice (or brown, but it will take longer)

1 tablespoon coconut or canola oil

4 cups cauliflower florets (14 ounces, or about ½ head)

¼ teaspoon kosher salt

1 15-ounce can chickpeas, rinsed and drained

1 12-ounce jar tikka masala simmer sauce (such as Maya Kaimal brand)

DRESS IT UP Chopped cilantro

1. Cook the rice according to the package directions.

2. Meanwhile, heat the coconut oil in a medium pot over medium-high heat. Add the cauliflower and salt and cook until the cauliflower is beginning to get tender, about 5 minutes.

3. Add the chickpeas and sauce. Bring to a simmer, cover, and cook until the cauliflower is tender, about 10 minutes. Serve over rice and top with cilantro, if using.

Ingredient Tip

Replace the cauliflower and/or chickpeas with 14 ounces extra-firm tofu, drained and diced.

Black Bean Burgers

MAKES 4 SERVINGS

Using refried beans is a shortcut to a delicious veggie burger—no additional seasoning required. I like squishy Martin's potato rolls for these patties.

1 14-ounce can refried black beans

1 large egg white

1 cup panko breadcrumbs

1 avocado, halved, pitted, and peeled

¼ teaspoon kosher salt

Juice of 1 lime

1 tablespoon canola or other neutral oil

4 burger buns

DRESS IT UP Hot sauce

1. In a medium bowl, combine the beans, egg white, and panko. Shape the mixture into 4 patties and place on a parchment-lined plate. Refrigerate for 15 minutes.

2. While the patties chill, mash the avocado, salt, and lime juice in a small bowl.

3. Heat the oil in a large nonstick skillet over medium heat. Cook the burgers until well browned, 3 to 4 minutes per side. Serve on the buns with the avocado mash; top with hot sauce, if desired.

ROUND IT OUT Any Green Leaf Salad (page 193), Quick Cukes (page 218), and/or Spicy Oven Fries (page 198)

Mediterranean Tuna Sandwiches

MAKES 4 SERVINGS

These easy-assembly, big-flavor sandwiches were my husband's discovery, and I am 100 percent on board. In my opinion, the anchovies are one of the best parts of this simple supper. But, if you aren't a fan, leave them out.

3 large eggs

½ cup pitted olives (such as Kalamata or Castelvetrano)

2 tablespoons mayonnaise

8 slices sandwich bread (preferably white bread), toasted and cooled

1 6–7-ounce jar tuna in olive oil, drained

8 anchovies

DRESS IT UP Baby arugula or basil leaves

1. Bring a medium pot of water to a boil. Carefully lower the eggs into the water, reduce the heat to a simmer, and cook for 11 minutes. Using a slotted spoon, transfer the eggs to a bowl of ice-cold water.

2. Peel and slice the eggs. Roughly chop the olives. Spread the mayonnaise on one side of each slice of cooled toast. Layer the tuna, olives, sliced egg, anchovies, and arugula or basil, if using, on 4 slices of the bread. Top with the remaining 4 slices. Press down on the sandwiches to help the filling hold together. Cut each sandwich in half and serve.

ROUND IT OUT Any Green Leaf Salad (page 193), Caprese-ish Salad (page 221), or Asparagus with Garlicky Mayo (page 210)

Moroccan-Spiced Tacos

MAKES 4 SERVINGS

Remember what I said at the beginning of this book about none of the recipes being authentic? This is an excellent example of that! Although this meaty filling is served wrapped in tortillas, it boasts a distinctly North African flair thanks to the toasty ras el hanout spice blend—a mix of cinnamon, cumin, and other warm spices—and the optional harissa sauce.

2 cups shredded cabbage (about 6 ounces)

Juice of ½ lemon (about 1 tablespoon)

1¼ teaspoons kosher salt, divided

2 tablespoons olive oil, divided

1 pound ground beef or ground lamb

1 tablespoon ras el hanout (sometimes labeled Moroccan spice blend)

1 tablespoon tomato paste

8 small flour tortillas, warmed

1 avocado, peeled, pitted, and sliced

DRESS IT UP Plain Greek yogurt, harissa

1. Combine the cabbage, lemon juice, and ½ teaspoon of the salt in a medium bowl. Toss with your clean hands, rubbing the salt into the cabbage. Let sit on the counter while you prepare the rest of the meal.

2. Heat 1 tablespoon of the olive oil in a large skillet over medium-high heat. Add the meat and cook, breaking it up with a spoon, until no longer pink. Drain in a colander in the sink, then return the meat to the pan.

3. Set the pan over medium heat. Add the remaining 1 tablespoon olive oil, remaining ¾ teaspoon salt, and ras el hanout. Cook, stirring, for 1 minute to toast the spices. Add the tomato paste and cook for another minute, stirring to make sure the meat is evenly coated. Add 2 tablespoons water, scraping up any spices or brown bits on the bottom of the pan. Remove the pan from the heat.

4. Serve the meat in the tortillas, topped with the avocado slices and some of the cabbage mixture. Garnish with yogurt and harissa, if desired.

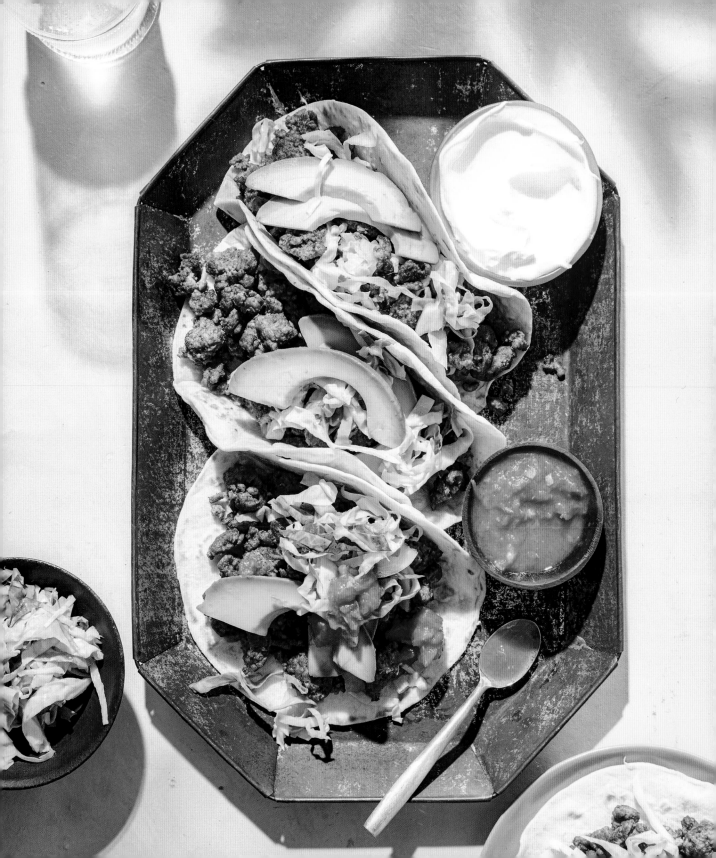

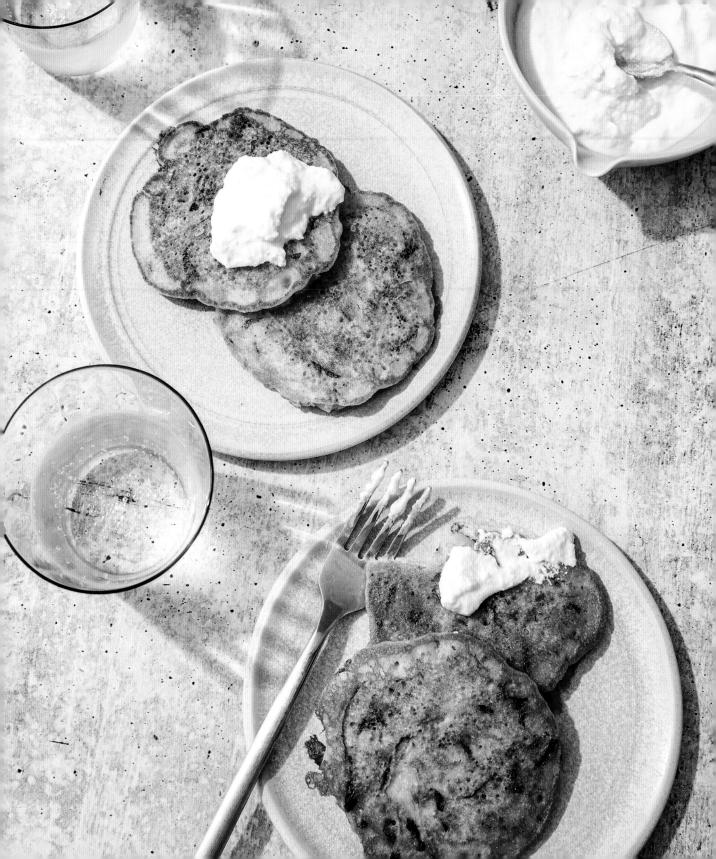

Zucchini-Herb Pancakes

MAKES 3 TO 4 SERVINGS

At one point as part of my job at Real Simple, *I found myself testing well over a dozen pancake mixes in my home kitchen. It hit me that I should take advantage of these practical mixes in my everyday cooking, and these surprisingly delicious pancakes were born. Use whatever combo of soft herbs you have; mint is especially lovely. While many mixes need only water, some require eggs, milk, or oil, so check the package directions before beginning the recipe.*

1 cup pancake mix (plus any eggs, milk, or oil the mix requires)

1 small zucchini, shredded (about 2 cups)

½ cup chopped soft herbs (such as parsley, mint, basil, tarragon, and/or cilantro)

½ teaspoon plus ⅛ teaspoon kosher salt, divided

½ teaspoon onion powder

Olive oil, for greasing the pan

¾ cup full-fat ricotta cheese

2 tablespoons milk

1 lemon

1. Prepare the pancake mix according to the package directions.

2. Wrap the shredded zucchini in a clean kitchen towel and squeeze it over the sink to wring out as much liquid as possible. Add the zucchini to the pancake batter along with the herbs, ½ teaspoon of the salt, and the onion powder.

3. Brush a griddle, nonstick skillet, or cast-iron skillet with olive oil and heat it over medium heat. Working in batches, drop ¼ cup of the batter for each pancake onto the pan. Cook until the pancakes are set and golden brown, 2 to 3 minutes per side. Gently press down on the pancakes with a spatula after flipping to flatten them slightly and help them cook all the way through.

4. Combine the ricotta, milk, and remaining ⅛ teaspoon salt in a small bowl. Zest the lemon into the bowl. Halve it and squeeze 2 teaspoons of the juice into the ricotta mixture. Stir and serve with the pancakes.

Spring Roll and Lettuce Roll-Ups

MAKES 4 SERVINGS

Is this the easiest recipe in the whole book? Maybe. It might also be one of the most delicious, since you basically get to eat appetizers for dinner. (Plus a lot of lettuce, so it totally counts as a real meal.)

2 pounds frozen mini spring rolls

1 head Bibb, red leaf, or green leaf lettuce

Sweet chili sauce, for serving (such as Taste of Thai)

DRESS IT UP Cilantro, basil, and/or mint leaves

Bake the spring rolls according to the package directions. Serve with a platter of lettuce leaves for wrapping at the table. Add herbs, if using. Dip in sweet chili sauce.

ROUND IT OUT Sesame-Soy Cauliflower Rice (page 208), Quick Cukes (page 218), or Quinoa Pilaf (page 222)

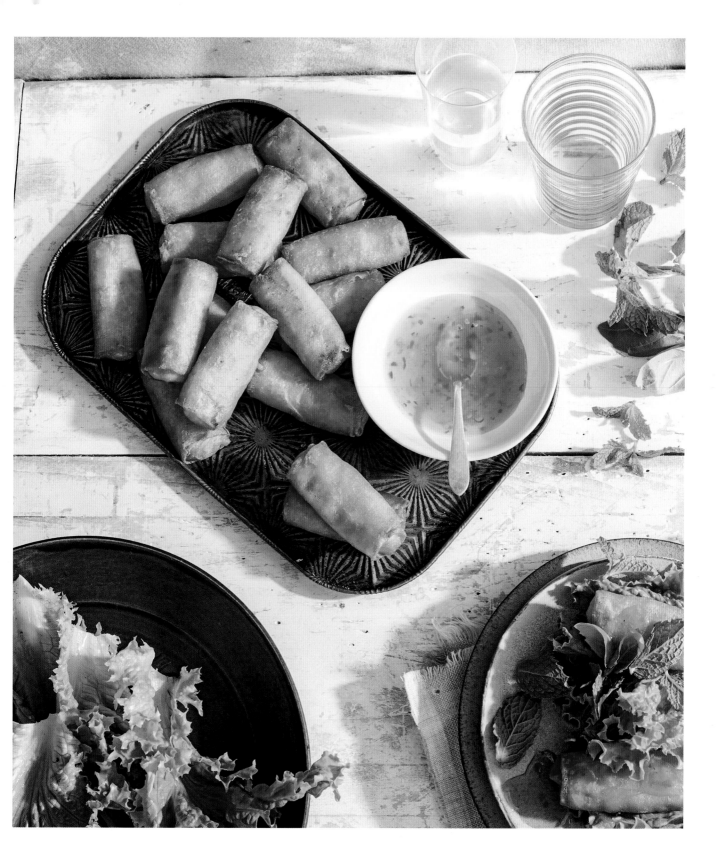

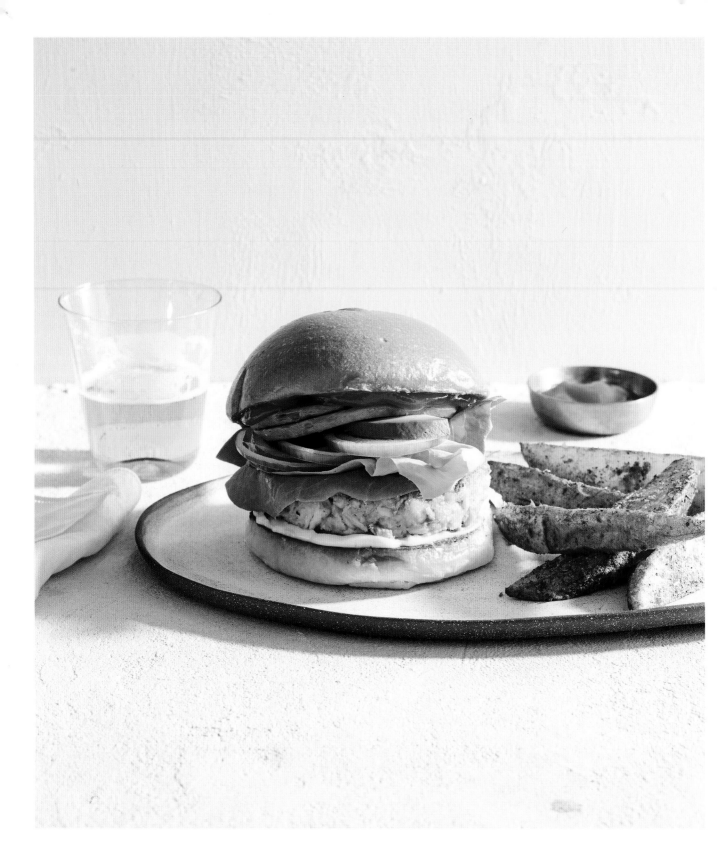

Shortcut Salmon Burgers

MAKES 4 SERVINGS

Canned salmon is a convenient and economical alternative to fresh, and it's ideal for easy burgers. Don't worry about any bones in the mix. When cooked, they become undetectable, and they are a source of calcium. I like to schmear these burgers with a combination of ketchup and mayo—delish.

15 ounces canned salmon, drained (2 to 3 cans)

½ cup panko breadcrumbs

¼ cup mayonnaise

2 teaspoons Dijon mustard

½ teaspoon kosher salt

Freshly ground black pepper to taste

1 tablespoon olive oil

4 burger buns (preferably brioche), toasted

Butter lettuce leaves, avocado slices, and sliced red onion, for serving

Ketchup and mayonnaise, for serving

1. Combine the salmon, panko, mayonnaise, mustard, salt, and pepper in a large bowl. Form into 4 patties and place on a parchment-lined plate. Refrigerate for 10 minutes.

2. Heat the olive oil in a large nonstick or cast-iron skillet. Cook the patties until golden brown, 2 to 3 minutes per side. Serve on the toasted buns with lettuce, avocado, red onion, ketchup, and mayonnaise.

ROUND IT OUT Spicy Oven Fries (page 198) and/or Eat-with-Everything Slaw (page 196)

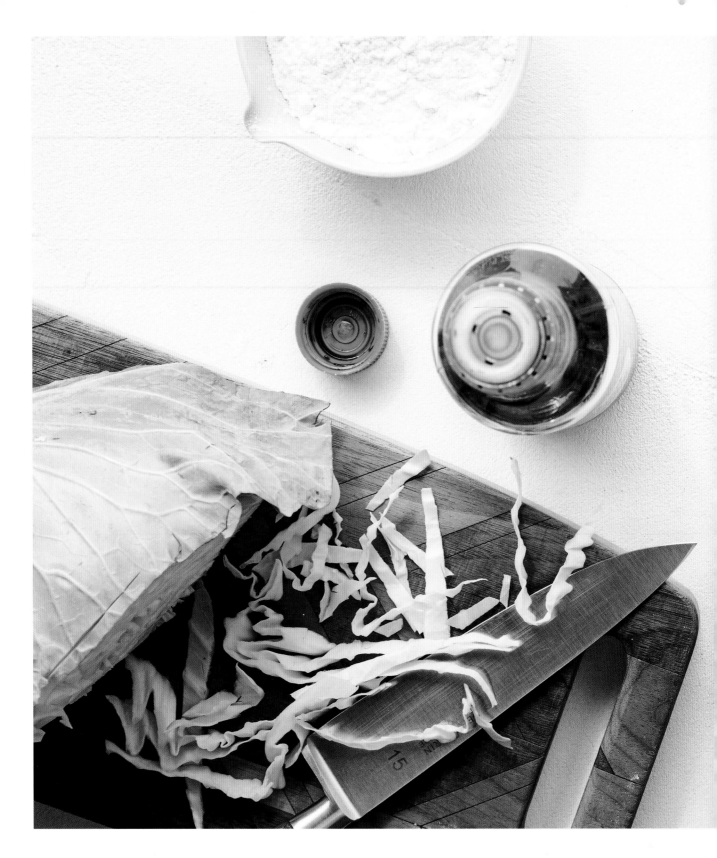

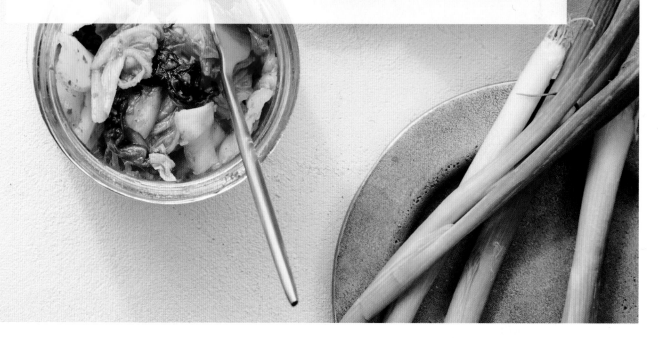

BARE MINIMUM
Ingredients

Recipes with Seven Ingredients (or Less)

Crispy Dijon Pork

MAKES 4 SERVINGS

This recipe features a couple of helpful shortcuts. First, instead of pounding the pork tenderloin into medallions, you can just press down with the heel of your hand. Will it be perfectly flat? Nope, and that's totally fine. Second, instead of dredging the pork in flour and then egg to get the breadcrumbs to adhere, coat the cutlets in Dijon mustard. The pork gets a boost of flavor and the panko gets something to hold on to.

2 tablespoons Dijon mustard

1 cup panko breadcrumbs

1 pork tenderloin, about 1 pound

¼ cup canola or other neutral oil (or for better flavor, use half neutral oil and half olive oil), plus more if necessary

Flaky sea salt to taste

1. Spoon the mustard into a small bowl and put the breadcrumbs in a shallow dish.

2. Cut the pork into 8 roughly equal rounds. Use the heel of your hand to press down on each cutlet, making it flattish. Using your fingers, smear the mustard all over the pork pieces. Then dredge the coated cutlets into the panko, pressing down to help the crumbs adhere.

3. Heat the oil in a large skillet over medium heat. Once the oil is hot, add as many pieces of pork as can fit in a single layer. Cook until golden brown, about 5 minutes per side. Transfer to a paper towel-lined plate to drain and sprinkle generously with flaky sea salt. If cooking a second batch, add another tablespoon or two of oil to the pan and cook the remaining pork.

ROUND IT OUT White Beans with Sage (page 202), Peas with Walnuts and Parm (page 213), or Roasted Shredded Brussels Sprouts (page 205)

Mushroom and Gruyère Quesadillas

MAKES 4 SERVINGS

I could eat quesadillas every day of the week, and I love to experiment with flavors that aren't quite traditionally Mexican. Here the Gruyère adds a nuttiness that plays well with the earthiness of the mushrooms.

1 15-ounce can refried black beans

2 tablespoons canola or other neutral oil, divided, plus more if necessary

4 ounces sliced mushrooms (such as cremini or a wild mushroom blend)

Pinch kosher salt

8 small corn tortillas

2 cups shredded Gruyère cheese (about 8 ounces)

DRESS IT UP Cholula or other hot sauce, sour cream

Ingredient Tip

Mushrooms are one of the few vegetables that you should season at the end of cooking, since the salt will draw out moisture and make it harder for them to brown.

1. Heat the refried beans in the microwave or on the stove-top. Keep warm.

2. Heat 1 tablespoon of the oil in a medium skillet. Add the mushrooms and cook until golden brown, about 5 minutes, stirring occasionally. Add a pinch of salt. Transfer to a small plate or bowl, reserving the skillet.

3. Place 4 tortillas on a work surface. Cover each with ¼ cup refried beans, then divide the mushrooms and cheese evenly over the beans (reserve the remaining refried beans for serving). Top with the remaining 4 tortillas.

4. Heat the remaining 1 tablespoon oil in the same skillet over medium-high heat. Cook the quesadillas one by one until crispy and golden, 1 to 2 minutes per side, adding more oil if necessary. Cut into quarters and serve with the remaining refried beans, plus the Cholula and/or sour cream if dressing it up.

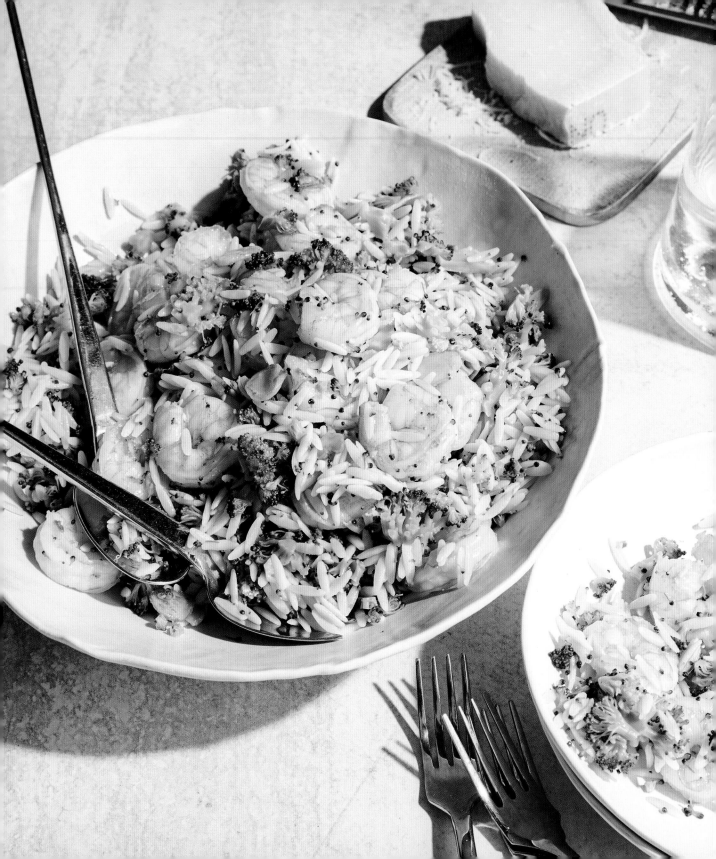

Broccoli and Shrimp Orzo

MAKES 4 SERVINGS

Since most shrimp at the fish counter has been previously frozen, it makes sense to buy frozen in the first place so there won't be any risk of the shrimp going bad in your fridge. To defrost, place the shrimp in a big bowl of cool water. After about 10 minutes, change the water. The shrimp will be thawed in about 20 minutes total (or less).

1¼ teaspoons kosher salt, divided, plus more for the pasta water

2–3 heads broccoli (about 1½ pounds)

⅓ cup olive oil, plus more for serving

3 cloves garlic, sliced

1 pound raw large shrimp (16–20 per pound), peeled and deveined

1 lemon, halved

12 ounces orzo (2 cups)

DRESS IT UP Crushed red pepper, grated Parmesan cheese

1. Preheat the oven to 400°F. Bring a large pot of well-salted water to a boil.

2. While the pasta water is coming to a boil, finely cut the broccoli florets off the stalks in about ¼-inch pieces, cutting from the floret end of each head. You should have about 4 cups. Reserve the stalks for another use. (I like to peel them and cut into sticks for snacking and dipping.)

3. Pour the olive oil into an 8 × 8-inch baking dish. Add the garlic and place in the oven for 5 minutes. Carefully remove the pan from the oven, add the shrimp and ½ teaspoon of the salt, and toss to coat. Return to the oven and cook for 9 to 10 minutes, until the shrimp are opaque. Squeeze one lemon half over the shrimp and stir.

4. While the shrimp are cooking, add the orzo to the boiling water and cook for 7 minutes. Add the chopped broccoli and cook for 2 more minutes. Drain and return to the pot.

5. Pour the shrimp mixture into the broccoli-orzo mixture, squeeze in the juice of the remaining lemon half, and add the remaining ¾ teaspoon salt; stir to combine. Serve, drizzled with more olive oil and dressed up with crushed red pepper and/or grated Parm, if desired.

Kimchi-Cabbage Cakes

MAKES 4 SERVINGS

I love okonomiyaki—large Japanese cabbage cakes made in a skillet and then cut into wedges to serve. But trust me, flipping one of those babies is not bare minimum. Instead, I make smaller cakes; they cook more quickly and are much (much!) easier to turn. Use a cast-iron skillet here if you have one.

6 cups shredded cabbage (preferably green; about 1 pound)

¾ cup chopped kimchi

4 scallions, trimmed and cut into 1-inch lengths

6 large eggs

3 tablespoons soy sauce or tamari

1 cup all-purpose flour

4 tablespoons canola or other neutral oil, divided, plus more if necessary

DRESS IT UP Mayonnaise mixed with sriracha

1. In a large bowl, stir together the cabbage, kimchi, and scallions. In a medium bowl, whisk together the eggs and soy sauce. Add to the cabbage mixture and toss to combine. Stir in the flour.

2. Heat 2 tablespoons of the oil in a large skillet over medium heat. Working in batches, drop ¾ cup of the batter for each patty into the oil. Cook until golden brown, 3 to 4 minutes per side. Transfer to a paper towel-lined plate to drain, and repeat with the remaining oil and cabbage mixture. Serve with the sriracha mayo, if using.

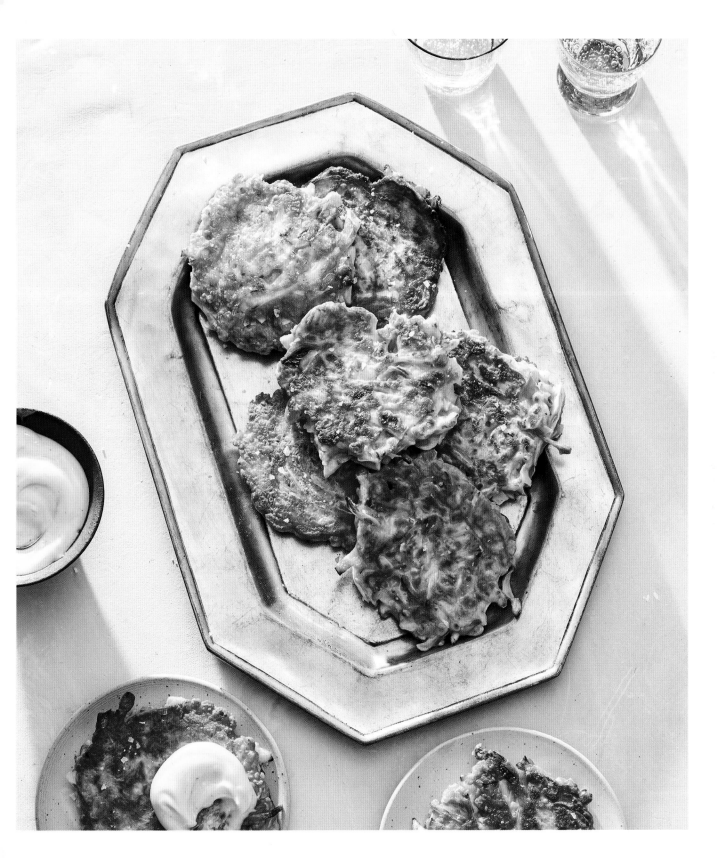

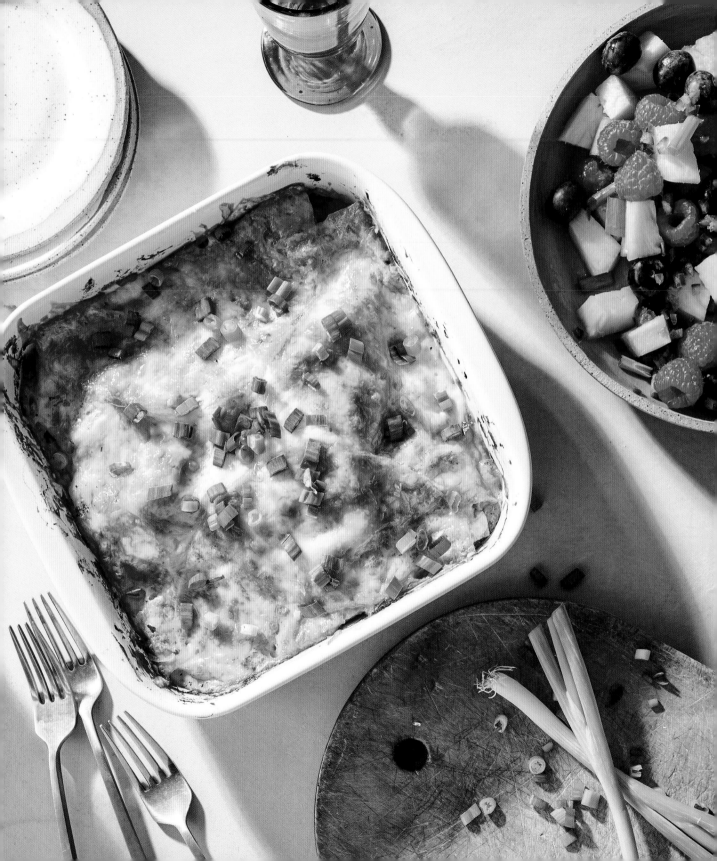

Chicken Enchilada Casserole

MAKES 4 SERVINGS

Rolling enchiladas is a worthy weekend project but not a bare minimum dinner, at least not at my house. This version provides all the pleasure of the original—the chew of the tortillas, the flavor of the sauce, and the creaminess of the cheese—in a free-form format.

2 cups shredded cooked chicken

1 cup enchilada sauce, divided

8 small corn tortillas

½ cup plain full-fat Greek yogurt, sour cream, or crème fraîche

1 cup shredded cheddar cheese (about 4 ounces)

1 scallion, trimmed and chopped

1. Preheat the oven to 375°F.

2. In a small bowl, toss the chicken with ¼ cup of the enchilada sauce.

3. Spread another ¼ cup enchilada sauce in the bottom of an 8 × 8-inch baking dish. Top with 4 tortillas; they will overlap some. Top with the chicken mixture and the remaining 4 tortillas.

4. In the same bowl you used for the chicken, whisk together the remaining ½ cup enchilada sauce and the yogurt. Pour over the tortillas, then top with the cheese. Bake for about 30 minutes, until golden brown. Sprinkle with the scallion and serve.

ROUND IT OUT Any Green Leaf Salad (page 193), Eat-with-Everything Slaw (page 196), or Savory Fruit Salad (page 217)

Apple-Cheddar Dutch Baby

MAKES 4 OR 5 SERVINGS

This dish would be just as welcome on the brunch table as on the dinner table, and I wouldn't fault you for adding a little maple syrup—no matter which meal you serve it at.

4 tablespoons (½ stick) unsalted butter

2 apples (such as Honeycrisp), cored and sliced

1 teaspoon kosher salt, divided

8 large eggs

1 cup milk

1 cup all-purpose flour

1½ cups shredded cheddar cheese (preferably smoked or extra sharp; about 6 ounces)

1. Preheat the oven to 425°F.

2. Heat the butter in a 10-inch oven-safe skillet over medium heat. Once it's bubbling, add the apples and ¼ teaspoon of the salt. Cook, stirring occasionally, until the apples are just tender, 5 to 7 minutes.

3. While the apples cook, whisk together the eggs, milk, flour, and remaining ¾ teaspoon salt until mostly smooth. It's okay if a few small lumps remain.

4. Pour the egg mixture into the pan with the apples. Top with the shredded cheese. Transfer the pan to the oven and bake until puffed and golden, 20 to 25 minutes. Cut into wedges to serve.

ROUND IT OUT Any Green Leaf Salad (page 193) or Asparagus with Garlicky Mayo (page 210)

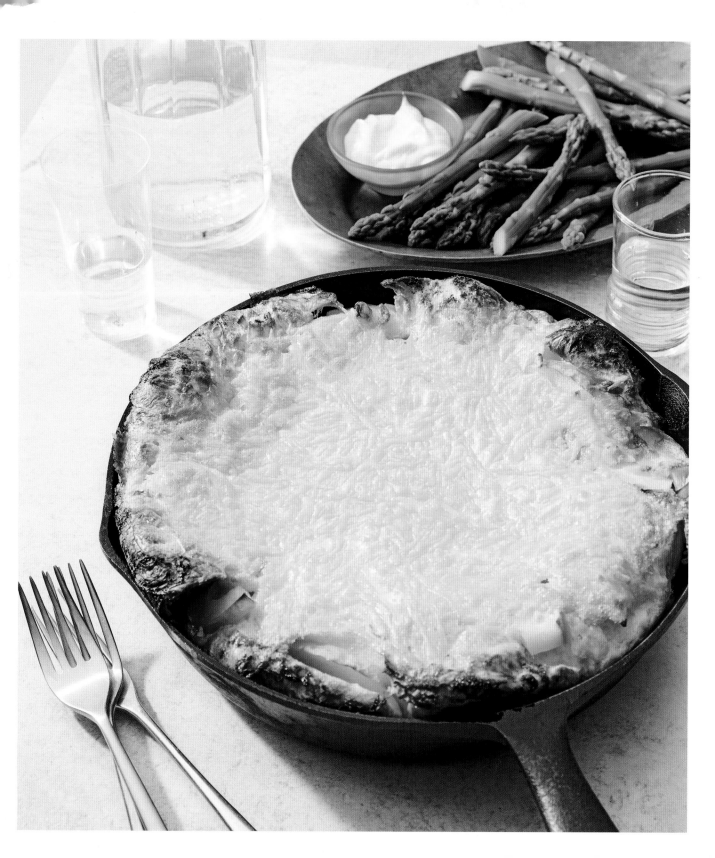

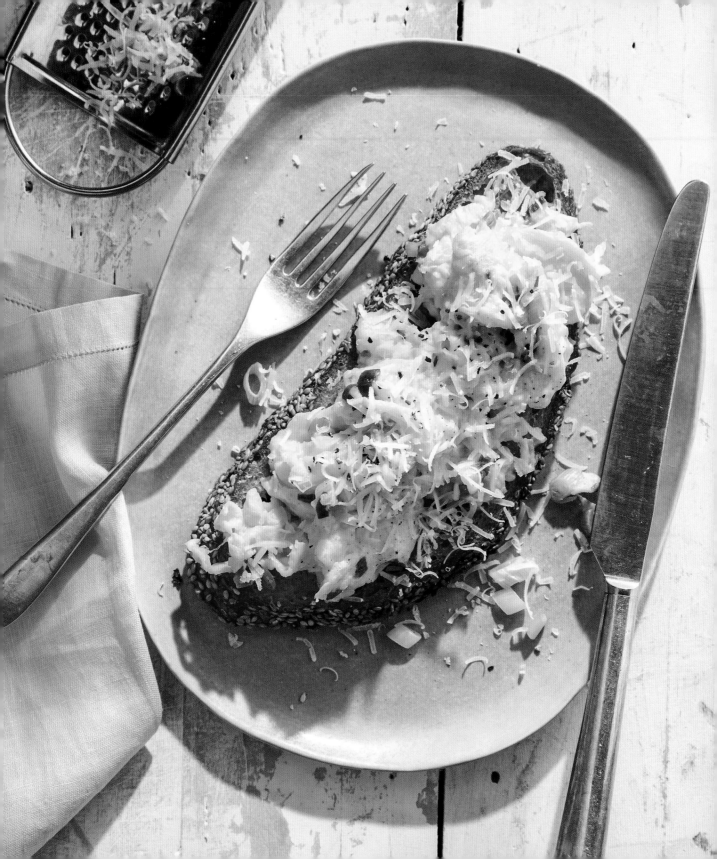

Eggs on Toast

MAKES 4 SERVINGS

A classic bare minimum dinner, this combo has seen my family through many a supper. Here are two of our favorite versions. They're also perfect for nights when you're eating on your own or with just one other person. Scale down the recipes as needed.

GUSSIED-UP EGGS ON TOAST

This is my teenager's recipe, and it's a meal I can completely endorse on a night you're craving a light supper. Use enough Parmesan for it to be totally irresistible.

1 tablespoon unsalted butter, plus more for the bread, divided

4 large slices bread or 8 smaller slices, toasted

8 large eggs

½ teaspoon kosher salt

2 scallions, trimmed and chopped

Grated Parmesan cheese and freshly ground black pepper, for serving

1. Butter the toast slices on one side.

2. Crack the eggs into a medium bowl. Add the salt, and whisk with a fork.

3. Heat the butter in a large nonstick pan over medium heat. Add the scallions and cook for 1 minute, stirring frequently. Add the eggs and scramble, stirring frequently. Spoon the cooked eggs over the buttered toast and top with plenty of Parmesan cheese and freshly ground black pepper to taste.

MISO AVOCADO TOAST WITH FRIED EGGS

You'll never want avocado toast without a miso boost again.

4 large slices bread, toasted

1 tablespoon olive oil, plus more for drizzling the toasts

2 avocados, pitted and peeled

2 tablespoons lemon juice

2 tablespoons white miso

4 large eggs

¼ teaspoon kosher salt

DRESS IT UP Sambal oelek or sriracha

1. Drizzle the toasts with olive oil and place on 4 plates.

2. Scoop the avocados into a medium bowl. Add the lemon juice and miso. Mash the avocado with a fork, making sure the miso is mixed in well. Spread on the toasts.

3. Heat the olive oil in a large nonstick pan over medium heat. Crack the eggs into the pan. Cover the pan and cook until the egg whites are just set, 3 to 4 minutes. Transfer 1 egg onto each avocado toast and sprinkle with the salt. Serve with sambal oelek or sriracha, if using.

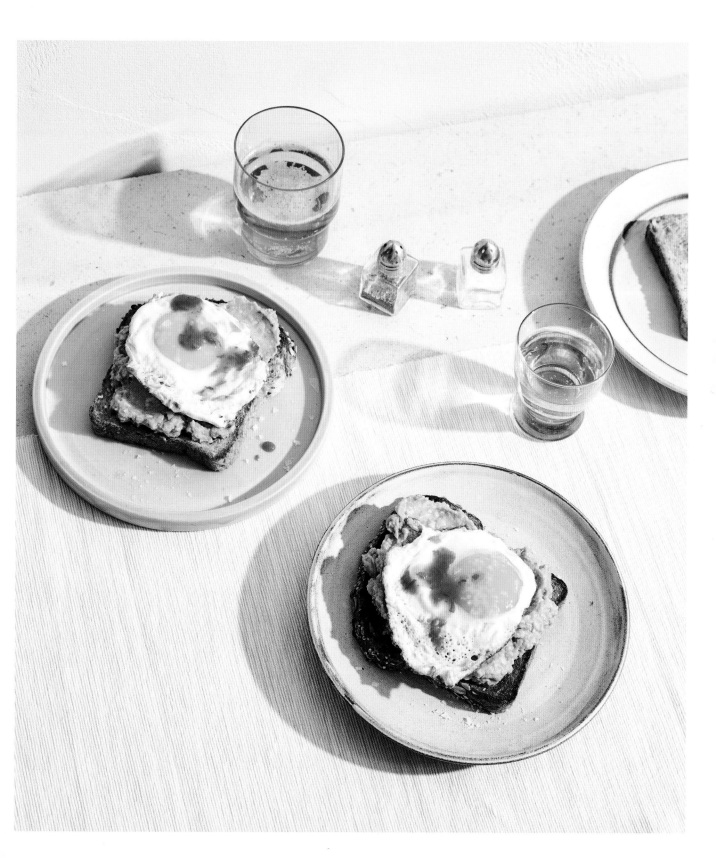

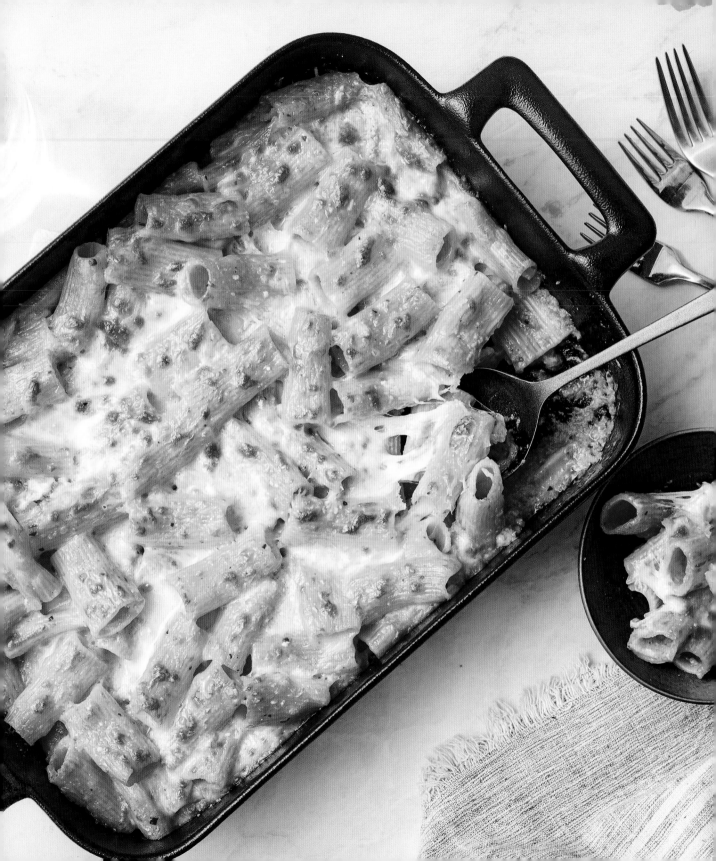

Baked Rigatoni

MAKES 6 SERVINGS

Traditional baked pastas like lasagna or baked ziti often feature either ricotta cheese or a homemade béchamel sauce added to tomato sauce. But, when I saw that cookbook author Julia Turshen uses crème fraîche instead, I was immediately smitten with the idea. It has a smoother texture and richer flavor than ricotta, and there's no need to make a separate sauce as you would with a béchamel. Penne or ziti will also work for this recipe. Just cook them 3 minutes short of al dente.

Olive oil, for greasing the pan

Kosher salt, for the pasta water

1 pound rigatoni

3 cups marinara sauce (24 ounces)

8 ounces crème fraîche

2 cups shredded low-moisture mozzarella cheese (about 8 ounces)

½ cup grated Parmesan cheese (about 2 ounces)

1. Preheat the oven to 375°F. Grease a 13 × 9-inch baking dish with olive oil.

2. Bring a large pot of salted water to a boil. Add the pasta and cook for 9 minutes. Drain and return the pasta to the pot. Stir in the marinara sauce and crème fraîche.

3. Transfer the pasta mixture to the prepared baking dish. Top with the mozzarella and Parmesan. Bake for about 30 minutes, until golden and bubbling. Let sit for 5 to 10 minutes before serving.

ROUND IT OUT Any Green Leaf Salad (page 193) or Everyday Broccoli (page 197)

Cooking Tip

Defrost a 10-ounce package of frozen spinach, squeeze out as much water as possible, and stir into the pasta and sauce mixture before transferring to the baking dish. Instead of spinach—or in addition—stir in 8 ounces of crumbled and cooked Italian sausage.

Balsamic-Soy Strip Steaks

MAKES 4 SERVINGS

This flavor combo may seem a little retro, but it was popular for a reason. The balsamic brings acid and sweetness to the party, while soy sauce adds a pop of saltiness and umami. They're the reason you can have so few ingredients in a marinade yet still end up with a flavor bomb of beef. Strip steaks are what I like to call weeknight steaks, under a half pound each and thin enough to cook quickly. Cook them on a grill pan as I call for here, in a cast-iron pan, or on a real grill outside.

2 tablespoons canola or other neutral oil, plus more for the pan

2 tablespoons balsamic vinegar

2 tablespoons soy sauce or tamari

4 ½-inch-thick strip steaks (about 1¾ pounds total)

Flaky sea salt to taste (optional)

ROUND IT OUT Spicy Oven Fries (page 198), Peels-On Cumin-Roasted Carrots (page 201), and/ or Fennel-Roasted Cabbage (page 214)

1. In a large, shallow dish, whisk together the oil, balsamic vinegar, and soy sauce. Add the steaks, turning to coat with a fork. Marinate for as little as 10 minutes or as long as 8 hours (cover and refrigerate if marinating for longer than 30 minutes). Turn the steaks once or twice while marinating.

2. Heat a grill pan over medium-high heat. Brush with oil. Grill the steaks for about 3 minutes per side for medium, or until they reach your desired level of doneness, cooking in batches if necessary depending on the size of your pan. Transfer to a plate and cover loosely with aluminum foil to keep warm. Let rest for 5 minutes.

3. Slice the steaks and put on plates. Pour any liquid from where the steaks rested over the sliced meat. Serve with a sprinkle of flaky sea salt, if desired.

Dead-Simple Sausage Soup

The flavor of this one-pot supper is really dependent on how delicious the sausage is. I prefer Aidells brand, but use your particular favorite.

1 tablespoon olive oil, plus more for drizzling

2 fully cooked chicken sausages (6–8 ounces), halved lengthwise and sliced crosswise

2 cups chicken broth

1 15-ounce can cannellini beans, rinsed and drained

1 14-ounce can diced tomatoes, with their juice

3 cups loosely packed baby spinach or baby arugula (about 1½ ounces)

1. Heat the olive oil in a medium pot over medium heat. Add the sausages and cook, stirring often, until browned, 3 to 5 minutes.

2. Add the broth, scraping up any brown bits from the bottom of the pan. Add the beans and tomatoes. Simmer for 5 minutes. Stir in the spinach or arugula. Divide into 4 bowls and serve topped with another drizzle of olive oil.

Grilled Ham and Cheese

MAKES 2 SANDWICHES

You may have heard of spreading mayonnaise on the outside of a grilled cheese instead of butter for an especially crispy sandwich. That's the idea here, except instead of spreading the mayo, I drop it straight into the pan to use it as the cooking fat. The bread still gets golden, and you can skip the spreading step.

4 slices bread

Dijon mustard, for spreading

1 cup grated sharp cheddar cheese (about 4 ounces)

4 thin slices ham (I like French ham, sliced paper-thin)

1 Bosc pear or apple, cored and thinly sliced

2 tablespoons mayonnaise

1. Lay the bread on a cutting board or work surface. Spread mustard on one side of each slice. Divide the cheese between 2 slices of bread. Top each with 1 slice of ham and then 2 or 3 pear or apple slices. (Serve the remaining fruit on the side.) Place the remaining bread on top of the sandwiches, mustard-side down.

2. Heat the mayonnaise in a large skillet over medium-high heat, breaking it up with a spoon until it's mostly melted. Add the sandwiches and cook until brown and crisp on the first side, about 3 minutes. Flip the sandwiches and reduce the heat to medium. Cook until the second side is golden and crispy and the cheese is melted, another 2 to 3 minutes.

ROUND IT OUT **Any Green Leaf Salad (page 193), Eat-with-Everything Slaw (page 196), or Everyday Broccoli (page 197)**

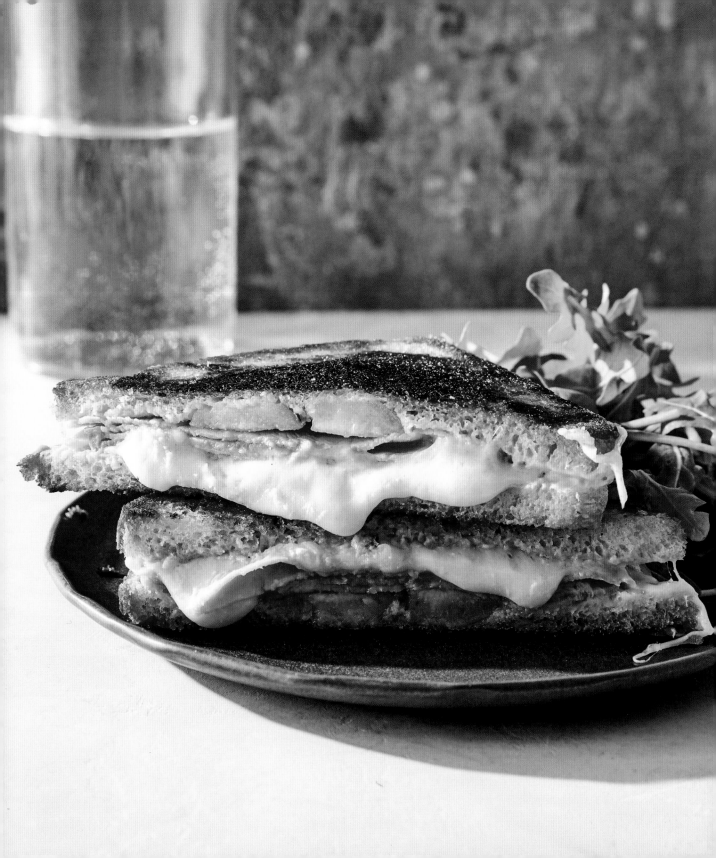

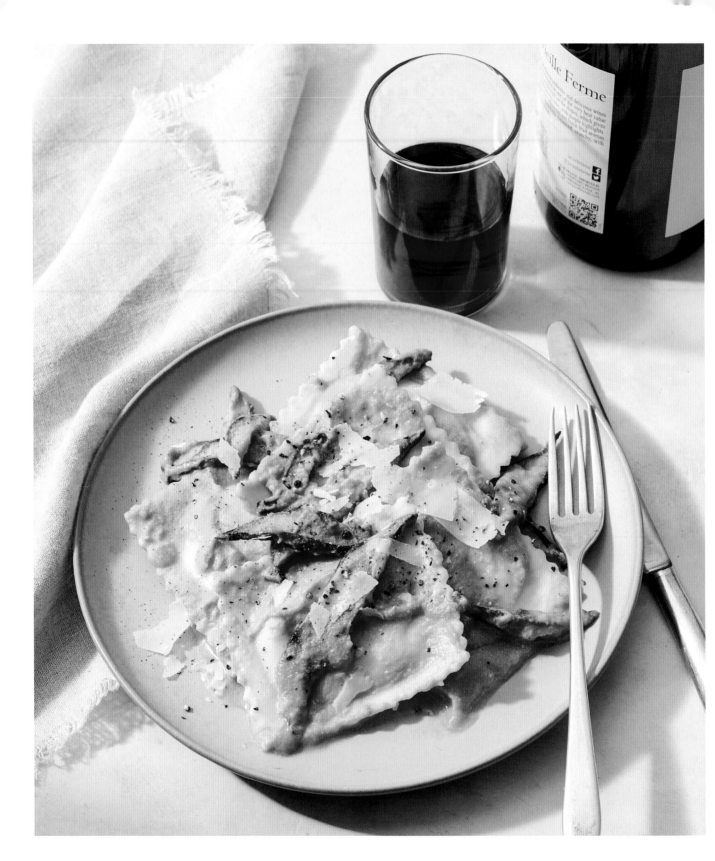

Pumpkin-Shiitake Ravioli

MAKES 4 SERVINGS

Store-bought vegetable broth is not quite as reliably consistent across brands as chicken broth. I think of some boxes (like Pacific and Imagine brands) as "orange" broths because they're heavy on the carrots. Other brands (like Kitchen Basics and Swanson) are more of a muddy green color. In a pinch, you can tell by looking at the photo on the boxes. Both orange and green have their uses; here you want to reach for an orange broth so it melds well with the pumpkin.

¾ teaspoon kosher salt, divided, plus more for the pasta water

1½ pounds cheese ravioli (refrigerated or frozen)

2 tablespoons olive oil

7 ounces shiitake mushrooms, stems discarded and caps thinly sliced

1 cup vegetable broth

½ cup canned pumpkin puree

½ cup half-and-half

DRESS IT UP Grated Parmesan cheese

1. Bring a large pot of salted water to a boil. Cook the ravioli according to the package directions. Drain and return to the pot.

2. Meanwhile, heat the olive oil in a large skillet or sauté pan over medium heat. Add the mushrooms and cook until golden brown, 8 to 10 minutes. Stir in ¼ teaspoon of the salt, then transfer the mushrooms to a bowl.

3. Add the broth to the pan and increase the heat to medium-high. Use a wooden spoon to scrape up any brown bits from the bottom of the pan. Whisk in the pumpkin and the remaining ½ teaspoon salt. Return the mushrooms to the pan and simmer for 3 minutes. Add the half-and-half and simmer for another minute.

4. Pour the sauce over the drained ravioli. Gently toss to coat. Serve with grated Parm, if desired.

BARE MINIMUM *Ingredients*

BBQ Pork Burgers and
Sweet Potato Fries

MAKES 4 SERVINGS

*Barbecue sauce is my teenager's favorite condiment, and we find lots of ways to
incorporate it into dinner. Of course, you can serve any side here, but sweet potato
fries go especially well.*

1 16–20-ounce bag frozen sweet potato fries (such as Alexia brand)

Canola or another neutral oil, for greasing the pan

1 yellow onion, sliced into rings

1 teaspoon kosher salt, plus more for the onions

1 pound ground pork

4 burger buns

Barbecue sauce, for serving

1. Cook the sweet potato fries according to the package directions. Keep warm in the oven while you prepare the rest of the dinner.

2. Brush a grill pan with oil and heat over medium heat. Add the onion rings and cook until softened with grill marks, about 5 minutes per side. Transfer to a plate and sprinkle with salt.

3. Combine the pork and 1 teaspoon salt in a medium bowl. Form into 4 patties.

4. Raise the heat to medium-high and place the patties on the grill pan. Cook until the interior of the burgers reaches 165°F on an instant-read thermometer, 4 to 5 minutes per side. Serve the burgers on the buns, topped with the onions and barbecue sauce, with the sweet potato fries on the side.

ROUND IT OUT Any Green Leaf Salad (page 193)

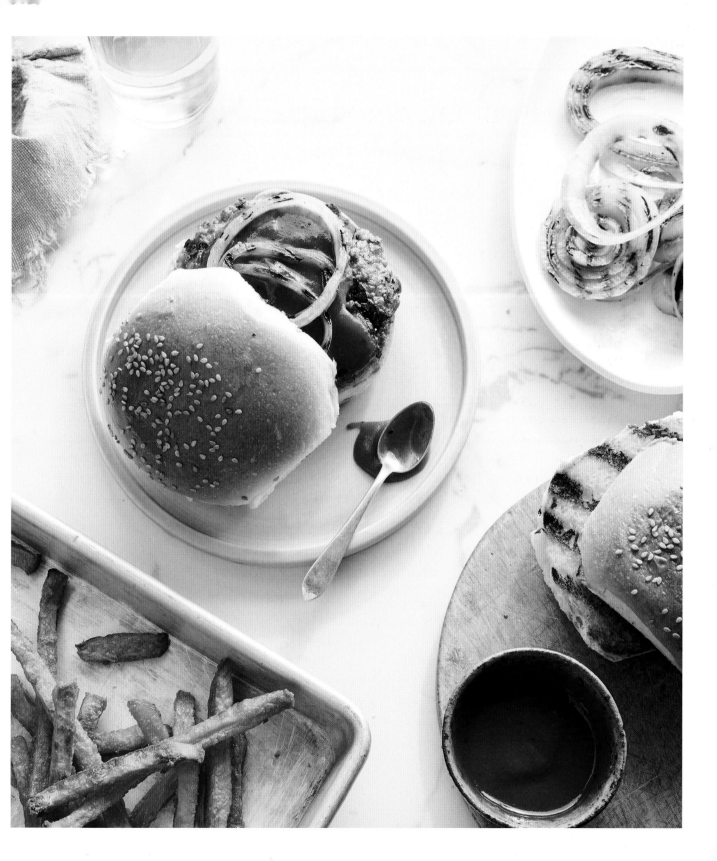

Kimchi and Pineapple Fried Rice

MAKES 4 SERVINGS

Store-bought baked tofu is a terrific shortcut in place of pressing and baking your own. Either plain or teriyaki varieties work well here. If you want to veg this up more, add a cup of sliced cabbage before the rice.

2 tablespoons canola or other neutral oil

4 cups cold cooked rice

1 cup chopped kimchi

7 ounces baked tofu, cut into 1 × ½-inch slabs

3 tablespoons soy sauce or tamari

1 cup chopped pineapple (small pieces)

¾ cup chopped cashews

DRESS IT UP Chopped cilantro, chopped scallions

1. Heat the oil in a very large nonstick or cast-iron pan or wok over medium-high heat. Add the rice and cook, stirring frequently, until beginning to crisp up, about 3 minutes.

2. Add the kimchi and tofu; stir and cook for 1 minute. Add the soy sauce; stir and cook for another minute. Stir in the pineapple and cashews and cook until warmed through. Serve topped with the cilantro and/or scallions, if using.

MAKE IT MEATY Omit the oil and cook 4 slices of bacon (or 4 ounces finely chopped pancetta) in the pan in step 1. Transfer the bacon to a paper towel–lined plate. Cook the rice in the bacon fat, then crumble the bacon and stir it in with the pineapple in step 2. Or, if you're serving both vegetarians and meat eaters, prepare the recipe as directed and cook the bacon or pancetta in a separate pan. Top the omnivores' portions with the meat.

Simple Tomato Soup

MAKES 4 SERVINGS

It doesn't get more comforting—or for me, nostalgic—than this. Serve with plenty of toast or crackers for dunking. If you have the ingredients, make a double batch and freeze the rest for a night when you could use a break.

2 tablespoons olive oil

1 yellow onion, chopped

1 28-ounce can crushed tomatoes

1 medium russet potato, peeled and chopped

1 teaspoon kosher salt

1 teaspoon balsamic vinegar

2 tablespoons unsalted butter

1. Heat the olive oil in a large pot over medium-high heat. Add the onion, reduce the heat to medium-low, and cook, stirring occasionally, until very tender, about 10 minutes.

2. Add the tomatoes, 2 cups water, potato, and salt. Bring the soup to a boil, reduce to a simmer, and cook until the potato is tender, 15 to 20 minutes. Cool for a few minutes.

3. With an immersion blender, puree the soup directly in the pot. Or, transfer the soup to a countertop blender and blend until smooth. (Always use caution when blending hot liquids: Remove the plastic insert from the lid, and cover the hole with a towel while blending.)

4. Stir in the vinegar and butter until melted.

ROUND IT OUT **Crusty bread, toast, or crackers; Any Green Leaf Salad (page 193)**

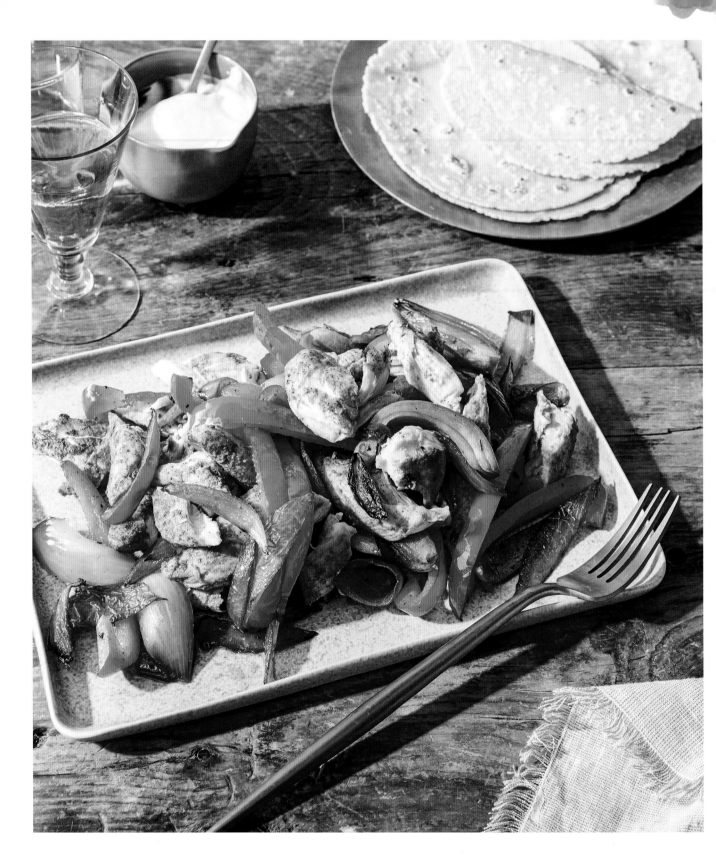

Chicken Tender Fajitas

MAKES 4 SERVINGS

Chicken tenders are a real time-saver here: They cook more quickly than breasts, and you don't need to slice them after they're cooked. If you have a cast-iron pan, use it for this recipe, since you can get it really hot for a great sear on the meat and veggies. Stainless will work too, but don't try this in nonstick. You won't be able to heat the pan enough to get that delicious browning.

2 tablespoons canola or other neutral oil, divided

1 pound chicken tenders

1 tablespoon fajita seasoning

2 large bell peppers, seeded and sliced

1 large red onion, cut into 16 wedges

1 teaspoon kosher salt

8 small flour or corn tortillas, warmed

DRESS IT UP Sour cream or plain Greek yogurt

V MAKE IT MEATLESS Swap out the chicken for 8 ounces sliced cremini mushroom caps. Cook until golden brown, about 5 minutes, then add the fajita spice blend. Cook for another minute, transfer the mushrooms to a bowl, and then continue with the recipe as written.

1. Heat 1 tablespoon of the oil in a large skillet or sauté pan over medium-high heat. Add the chicken and fajita seasoning. Toss with tongs until all the tenders are coated, then spread them out in a single layer. Cook for 3 minutes, then flip each tender. Continue cooking until the chicken is cooked all the way through, about 3 more minutes. Transfer the chicken to a plate.

2. Reduce the heat to medium. Add the remaining 1 tablespoon oil, peppers, onion wedges, and salt. Cook, tossing occasionally, until well browned and tender-crisp, about 10 minutes. Add ¼ cup water and use a wooden spoon to scrape up and incorporate any brown bits on the bottom of the pan.

3. Tear each tender into 3 or 4 pieces and return to the pan, along with any accumulated juices on the plate. Toss to combine. Serve in the tortillas with sour cream or yogurt, if desired.

Farro and Tuna Salad

MAKES 4 SERVINGS

Giardiniera is a mix of Italian-style pickled vegetables; you can find jars near the pickles in most supermarkets. Some versions will be spicy, others just tangy. Use it liberally to perk up sandwiches, pasta, or hearty grain salads like this one. You don't need to dress the greens separately here; the seasonings from the salad will do the job for you.

¾ teaspoon kosher salt, plus more for cooking the farro

1 cup uncooked farro (2½ cups cooked)

2 cups chopped giardiniera

3 tablespoons olive oil

1 6–7-ounce jar tuna in olive oil, drained

4 cups loosely packed leafy greens (such as baby spinach or baby arugula; about 2 ounces)

Freshly ground black pepper to taste

1. Cook the farro in well-salted water according to the package directions. Drain and transfer to a large bowl. Let cool for 10 to 15 minutes, stirring occasionally to help the steam escape.

2. Stir the giardiniera, olive oil, and salt into the farro. Gently stir in the tuna.

3. Divide the greens among 4 shallow bowls. Top with the farro mixture and plenty of pepper.

V MAKE IT MEATLESS **Replace the tuna with 4 hard-boiled eggs, sliced.**

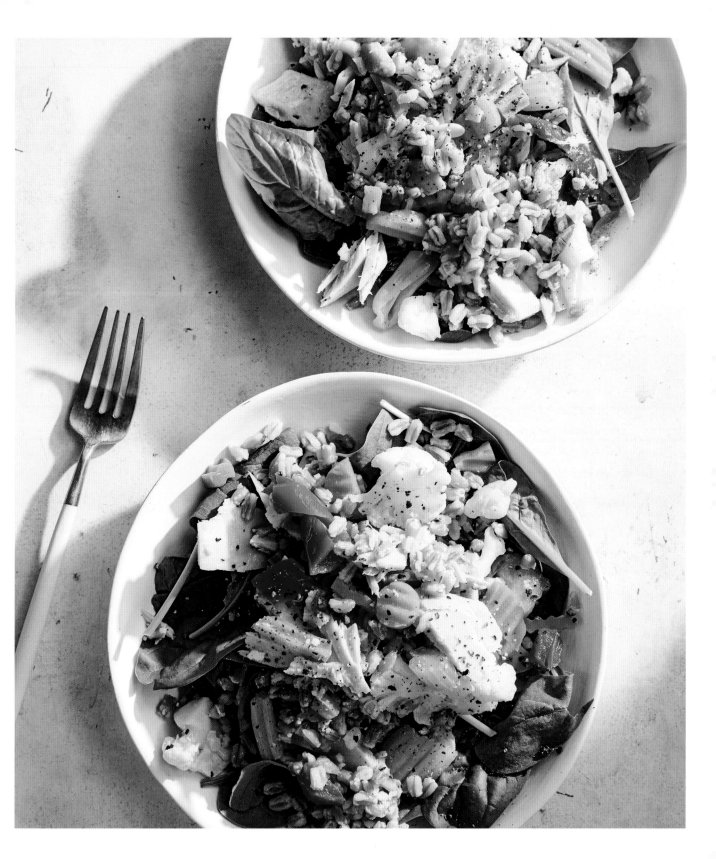

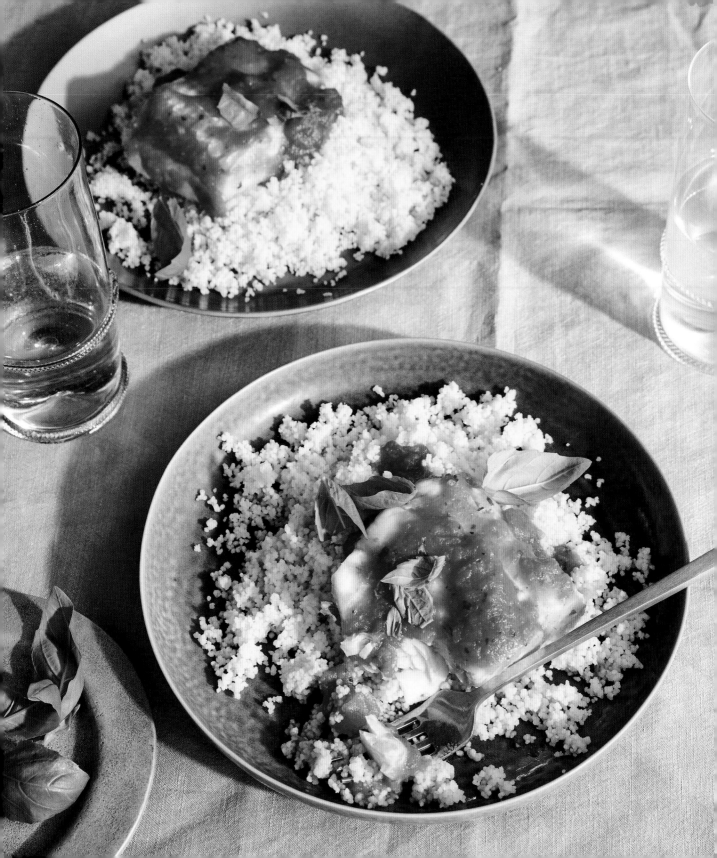

Marinara-Poached Cod

MAKES 4 SERVINGS

Marinara sauce is more than just a topping for pasta. In this recipe, it acts as a poaching liquid for fish. Serve this ultra-simple meal over a starch to soak up the sauce.

Orzo, rice, couscous, or instant polenta (enough for 4 servings)

2 cups marinara sauce

½ teaspoon kosher salt

4 5-ounce cod fillets

2 tablespoons unsalted butter

DRESS IT UP Torn basil leaves

1. Cook your choice of starch according to the package directions. Keep warm.

2. In the meantime, bring the marinara to a simmer in a medium nonstick skillet over medium heat. Sprinkle the salt on both sides of the cod fillets and nestle the fish into the marinara. Cover and simmer until the cod is just cooked through, about 15 minutes depending on the thickness of the fillets.

3. Divide the starch into 4 shallow serving bowls. Top with the fish, leaving most of the marinara behind in the skillet.

4. Stir the butter into the marinara until melted. Pour the sauce over the fish and serve, topping with torn basil leaves, if desired.

ROUND IT OUT Any Green Leaf Salad (page 193), Everyday Broccoli (page 197), or Fennel-Roasted Cabbage (page 214)

BARE MINIMUM *Ingredients*

Whole-Wheat Pasta with Chard and Garlic

MAKES 4 SERVINGS

This is one of the few recipes in this book where I call specifically for whole-wheat pasta (although, of course, you can swap it in elsewhere—or swap it out here!). I love the heartiness, flavor, and chew of whole-wheat in this simple dish. And don't be afraid of the anchovies! No one will know they're there, but they add a savory richness to the meal. If the chard is ready before the spaghetti, just turn the heat to low while you wait for the pasta to finish cooking.

¼ teaspoon kosher salt, plus more for the pasta water

12 ounces whole-wheat spaghetti

2 bunches Swiss chard

3 tablespoons olive oil, plus more for serving

3 anchovy fillets

3 cloves garlic, sliced

½ cup toasted pine nuts or chopped toasted walnuts or almonds

DRESS IT UP Crushed red pepper, flaky sea salt

V MAKE IT MEATLESS Omit the anchovies and don't forget the flaky salt.

1. Bring a large pot of well-salted water to a boil. Cook the pasta until al dente, 9 to 10 minutes. Do not drain.

2. Meanwhile, slice the stems out of the chard leaves and cut the stems into 2-inch lengths. Chop the leaves.

3. Heat the olive oil in a large sauté pan over medium heat. Add the anchovies and break them up with a spoon until they dissolve in the oil. Add the garlic and chard stems and cook until just tender, about 3 minutes. Add the chard leaves and salt. Cook, stirring, until the leaves start to wilt, about 3 minutes.

4. Using tongs, transfer the cooked pasta to the pan with the chard. Add enough pasta water to fully wilt the leaves. Toss the pasta with the leaves using tongs. Serve topped with the pine nuts, a drizzle of olive oil, and crushed red pepper and sea salt, if desired.

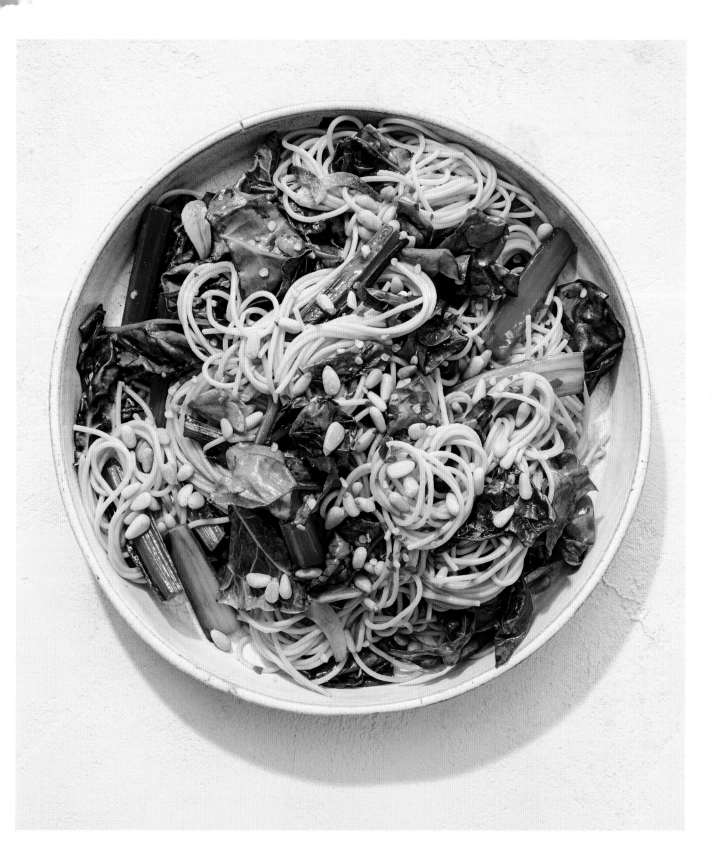

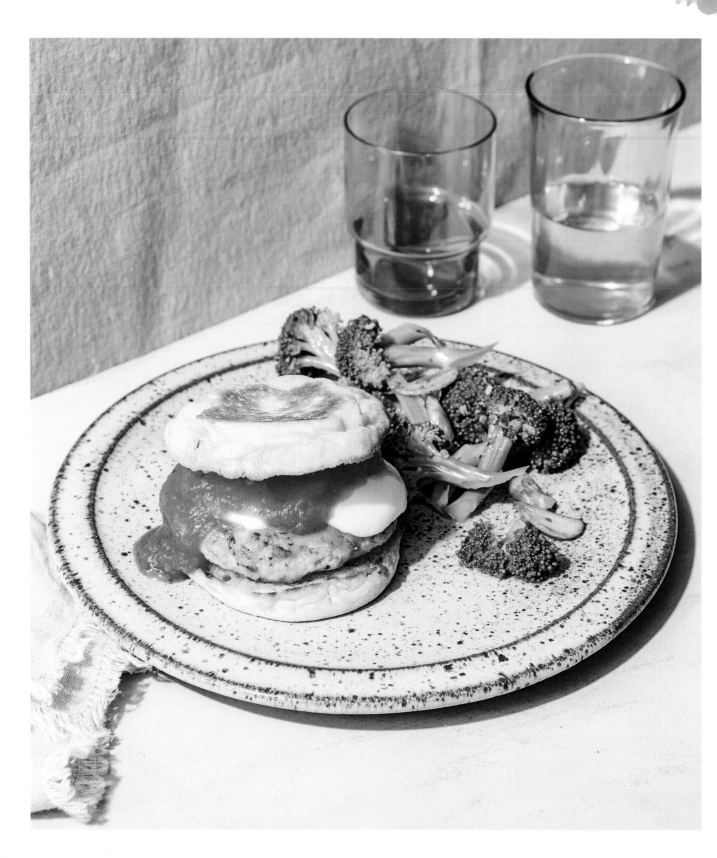

Chicken Parm Burgers

MAKES 4 SERVINGS

Savory chicken, bright tomato sauce, and gooey cheese all come together in these family-friendly burgers. While a brioche or potato bun is always a safe bet, I also like these burgers on toasted English muffins.

1 pound ground chicken (not all breast meat)

1½ teaspoons Italian seasoning

¾ teaspoon kosher salt

2 tablespoons olive oil

4 slices fresh mozzarella cheese (4 ounces)

1 cup marinara sauce, warmed

4 English muffins or burger buns, toasted

1. In a large bowl, mix together the ground chicken, Italian seasoning, and salt. Form into 4 patties.

2. Heat the olive oil in a large skillet over medium-high heat. Add the patties and cook until golden brown and nearly cooked through (about 150°F on an instant-read thermometer), about 6 minutes per side. Reduce the heat to medium, top each patty with a slice of cheese, cover the pan, and cook until the cheese is melted and the patties reach 165°F, about 3 minutes. Divide the marinara evenly over the patties and serve on the toasted English muffins.

ROUND IT OUT Any Green Leaf Salad (page 193), Everyday Broccoli (page 197), Spicy Oven Fries (page 198), or Fennel-Roasted Cabbage (page 214)

Bacon and Corn Frittata

MAKES 4 SERVINGS

Using frozen corn makes this dish super-convenient and delicious even in the dead of winter. But, if you have fresh, height-of-summer sweet corn, go for it! Cut the kernels off 3 ears and sauté them for 1 minute with the bacon before adding the egg mixture.

4 slices bacon

1 10-ounce package frozen corn, thawed and drained

2 scallions, trimmed and chopped

7 large eggs

⅓ cup whole milk, plain whole-milk yogurt, or buttermilk

¾ teaspoon kosher salt

Freshly ground black pepper to taste

1. Preheat the oven to 350°F.

2. Using kitchen shears, cut the bacon into 1-inch pieces directly into a 10-inch oven-safe skillet. Place over medium-high heat and cook, stirring occasionally, until the bacon is crisp, about 5 minutes. Stir in the corn and scallions.

3. In a medium bowl, whisk together the eggs, milk, salt, and pepper. Pour the egg mixture over the bacon-corn mixture and cook over medium heat for 3 minutes.

4. Transfer to the oven and bake until just set, 12 to 14 minutes. Let stand for at least 5 minutes before slicing and serving.

V MAKE IT MEATLESS Skip the bacon. In step 2, add 2 tablespoons olive oil to the pan. Sauté 4 ounces sliced shiitake mushrooms until crisp and golden, about 5 minutes. Sprinkle with a pinch of salt and continue with the recipe.

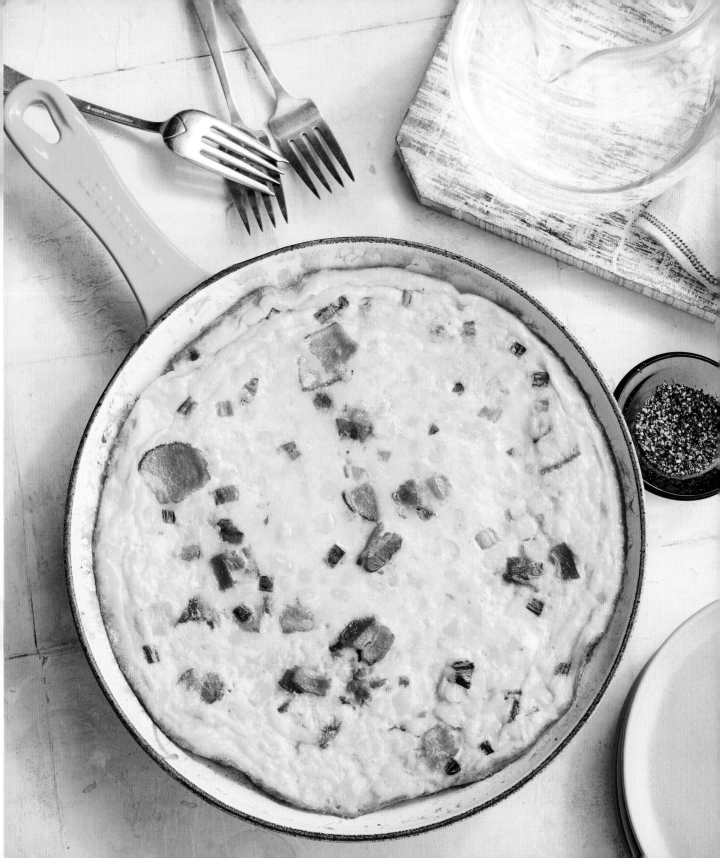

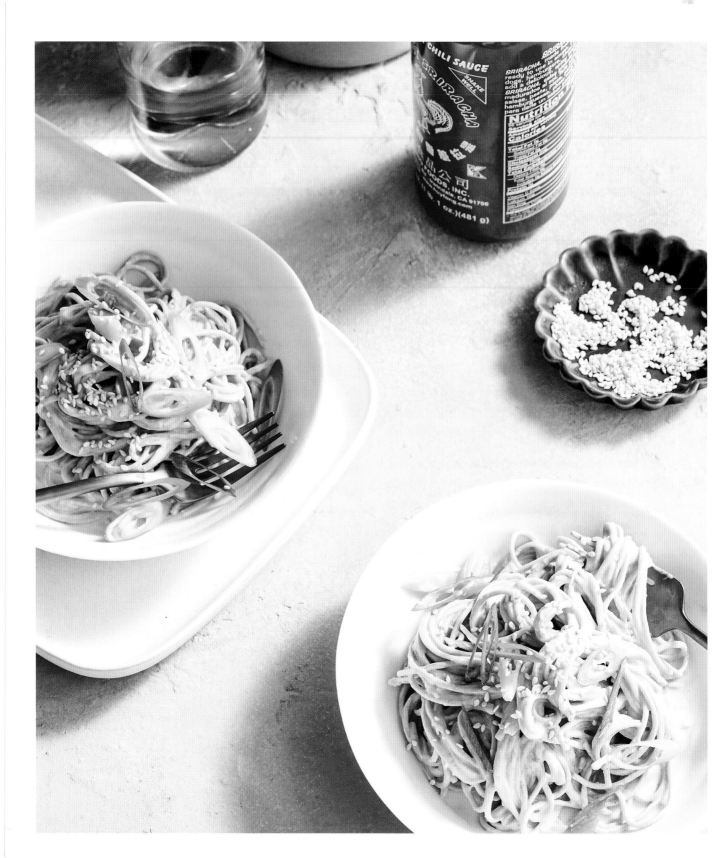

Tahini-Coconut Noodles

MAKES 4 SERVINGS

Leftover noodles are perfect for the lunch box.

Kosher salt, for the pasta water

⅓ cup tahini

⅓ cup canned coconut milk (well shaken)

3 tablespoons white miso paste

1½ tablespoons rice vinegar

1 tablespoon maple syrup

9 ounces soba noodles

DRESS IT UP Chopped scallions, toasted sesame seeds, sriracha or sambal oelek

1. Bring a medium pot of salted water to a boil. While it's heating up, whisk together the tahini, coconut milk, miso paste, rice vinegar, and maple syrup in a large bowl.

2. Once the water has come to a boil, cook the noodles according to the package directions, about 4 minutes. Drain, rinse with cold water, and drain again, shaking off excess water. Transfer to the bowl with the coconut-miso sauce. Toss with tongs to combine. Serve with scallions, sesame seeds, and/or hot sauce, if desired.

ROUND IT OUT Eat-with-Everything Slaw (page 196) and/or Quick Cukes (page 218)

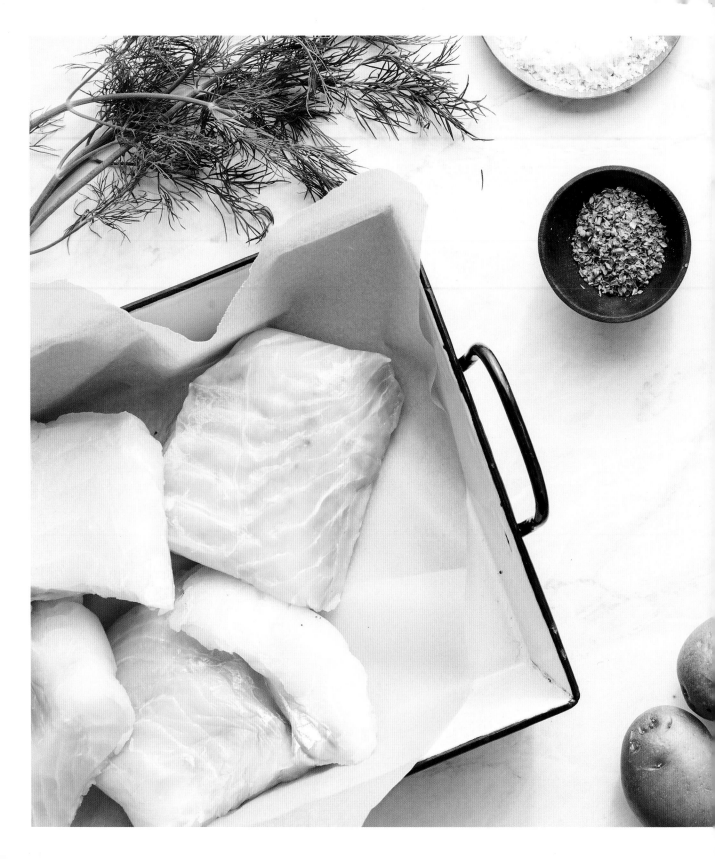

BARE MINIMUM
Cleanup

Dinners That Come Together in a Single Pot or Pan

Sesame-Maple Tofu Bake

MAKES 4 SERVINGS

A simple sweet-and-salty marinade of soy sauce, sesame oil, and maple syrup gives roasted tofu, sweet potatoes, and cauliflower big flavor.

1 14-ounce package extra-firm tofu

2 sweet potatoes, cut into chunks

4 cups cauliflower florets (about ½ head)

1 tablespoon canola or other neutral oil

1 teaspoon kosher salt

3 tablespoons soy sauce or tamari

3 tablespoons toasted sesame oil

2 tablespoons maple syrup

DRESS IT UP Roasted nori strips (aka seaweed snacks), toasted pepitas, roughly chopped cilantro, sriracha

1. Preheat the oven to 425°F.

2. Place the tofu on a paper towel–lined plate. Top with another paper towel and another plate. Place a box of broth or a can or tomatoes on the top plate to weight it down. Let the tofu drain for about 10 minutes while you get the veggies into the oven.

3. Line a rimmed baking sheet with parchment paper. Put the sweet potato chunks and cauliflower florets on the sheet. Drizzle with the oil and sprinkle with the salt. Toss to combine, then spread out in a single layer and roast for 20 minutes.

4. While the vegetables cook, whisk together the soy sauce, sesame oil, and maple syrup in a shallow dish. Cut the pressed tofu into 8 squares and put them in the sesame-soy mixture. Turn to coat. Let the tofu marinate, turning a few times, while the vegetables cook.

5. After the vegetables have cooked for 20 minutes, carefully remove the pan from the oven. Scoot the vegetables to the edges of the pan and place the tofu in the middle. Drizzle any remaining marinade over the vegetables and tofu. Roast for another 20 minutes.

6. Serve topped with nori, pepitas, cilantro, and/or sriracha, if desired.

Springy Chicken and Asparagus

MAKES 4 SERVINGS

Of course, you can eat this meal in summer, fall, or winter. But I get most excited about asparagus come spring, when its appearance at the farmers' market means that winter is really and truly over. It's also a lighter meal, ideal for warmer days.

4 tablespoons olive oil, divided, plus more if necessary

1 pound asparagus, woody ends snapped off

¾ teaspoon kosher salt, divided

1 pound thinly sliced chicken cutlets (4–6 cutlets)

Freshly ground black pepper to taste

¾ cup almond flour

Flaky sea salt to taste

1. Heat 1 tablespoon of the olive oil in a large skillet, preferably nonstick, over medium heat. Add the asparagus and ¼ teaspoon of the salt and cook for 3 minutes, using tongs to move the asparagus around occasionally. Add 2 tablespoons water. Cover and cook until just tender, about 2 minutes. Transfer the asparagus to a plate. Turn off the heat and wipe out the skillet.

2. Sprinkle the chicken cutlets on both sides with the remaining ½ teaspoon salt and plenty of pepper. Put the almond flour on a plate. Press each cutlet into the flour and place on a parchment-lined plate.

3. Heat another 2 tablespoons olive oil in the same skillet over medium heat. Add 2 cutlets (or more if the pan is large enough; do not crowd them). Cook until golden brown and cooked through, 2 to 3 minutes per side. Transfer to a plate and sprinkle with flaky sea salt. Repeat with the remaining 1 tablespoon olive oil, plus more if necessary, and remaining cutlets. Serve with the asparagus.

ROUND IT OUT Crusty bread, Quinoa Pilaf (page 222), or Spicy Oven Fries (page 198)

BARE MINIMUM *Cleanup*

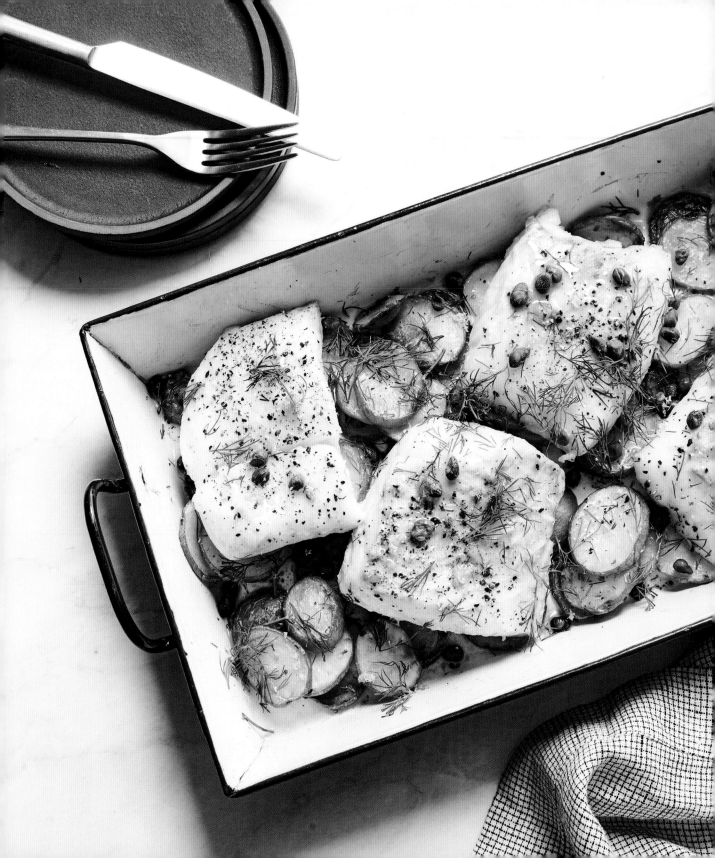

Lemony Cod and Potatoes

MAKES 4 SERVINGS

Cod is a mildly flavored fish, making it perfect for seafood skeptics. Be sure to cut the potatoes thinly, so they cook all the way through. No capers? Use chopped olives instead.

3 tablespoons olive oil, divided

2 pounds red potatoes, sliced ¼ inch thick

1½ teaspoons kosher salt, divided

¾ teaspoon dried oregano, divided

4 5–6-ounce cod fillets

Freshly ground black pepper to taste

1 lemon

1 tablespoon capers

DRESS IT UP Chopped dill

1. Preheat the oven to 400°F.

2. Pour 2 tablespoons of the olive oil into a 13 × 9-inch baking dish. Add the potatoes, 1 teaspoon of the salt, and ½ teaspoon of the oregano. Toss to combine, then spread out in a mostly single layer. Bake for 30 minutes.

3. Season the cod fillets on both sides with the remaining ½ teaspoon salt and a few grinds of pepper. Place the fish on top of the baked potato slices. Sprinkle the fish with the remaining ¼ teaspoon oregano and drizzle with the remaining 1 tablespoon olive oil. Zest the lemon over the fish and potatoes and sprinkle on the capers. Bake until the fish flakes easily with a fork, 12 to 15 minutes.

4. Cut the zested lemon in half and squeeze half over the fish and potatoes (reserve the other lemon half for another use). Serve the fish and potatoes topped with chopped dill, if desired.

ROUND IT OUT Any Green Leaf Salad (page 193), Everyday Broccoli (page 197), or Asparagus with Garlicky Mayo (page 210)

3 Skillet Egg Dinners

Eggs can be simmered in all manner of deliciousness on the stove-top—think eggs in purgatory or Israeli shakshuka—for simple one-pan dinners. Here are three of my favorite riffs on the technique.

SPICED BEANS AND EGGS

MAKES 4 SERVINGS

Jarred salsa adds instant flavor to beans.

½ cup thinly sliced red onion

2 tablespoons red wine vinegar

¼ teaspoon kosher salt, plus more for the eggs

2 15-ounce cans black beans, rinsed and drained

1 cup tomato salsa

4 large eggs

4 flour or corn tortillas, warmed

DRESS IT UP Chopped cilantro, sour cream or plain Greek yogurt

1. Combine the onion, vinegar, and salt in a small bowl. Let sit on the countertop to make a very quick pickle while you prep the rest of the meal.

2. Combine the beans, salsa, and ½ cup water in a large skillet. Bring to a simmer over medium heat and cook for 5 minutes.

3. Crack the eggs into the bean mixture. Cover and cook for 5 to 8 minutes, until the eggs are cooked to your liking. Season each egg with salt.

4. Scoop the beans and eggs into 4 shallow bowls and top with cilantro, if using. Serve with the tortillas, pickled red onion, and sour cream or yogurt, if desired.

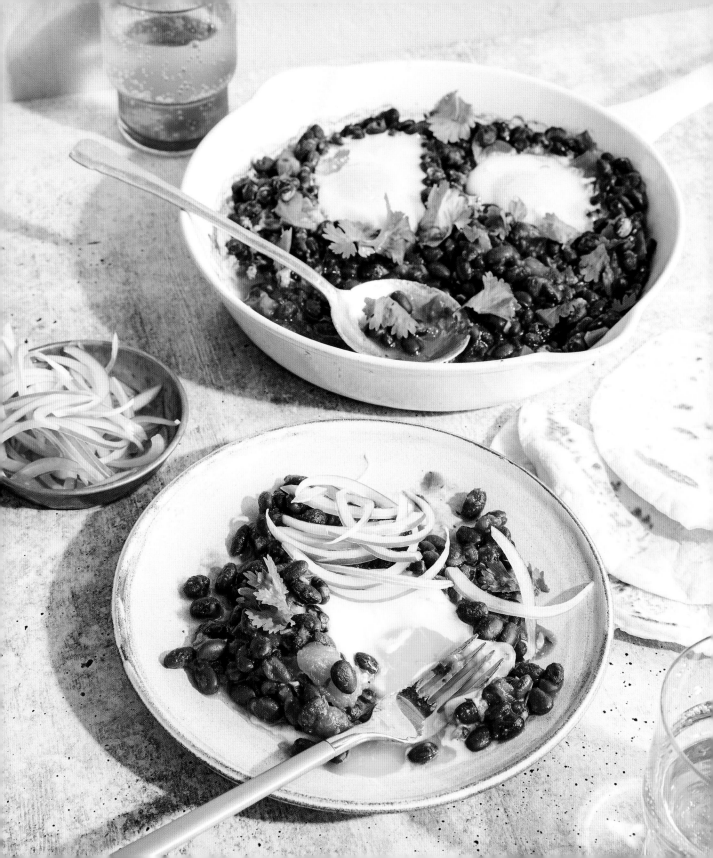

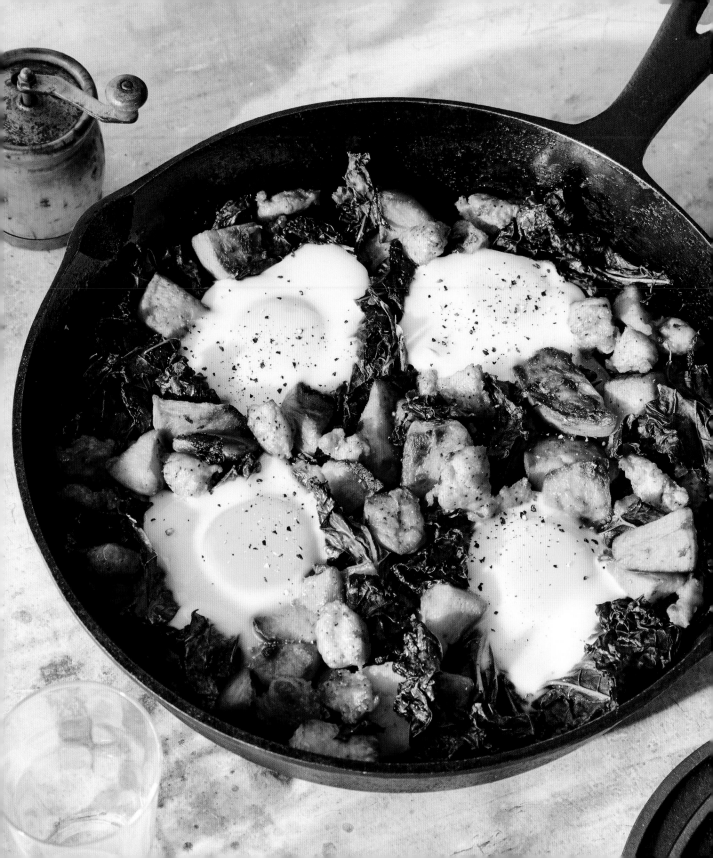

SWEET POTATO AND SAUSAGE HASH

MAKES 4 SERVINGS

This one-pot meal is made extra easy thanks to frozen fire-roasted sweet potato chunks. (I buy Cascadian Farm brand.) If your fam prefers regular white spuds, feel free to use those instead.

3 tablespoons olive oil, divided

8 ounces sweet or hot Italian sausage, removed from its casings

1 bunch curly kale, stems removed and leaves torn into pieces, washed but not dried (about 10 cups)

½ teaspoon kosher salt, divided

1 1-pound bag frozen fire-roasted sweet potatoes

4 large eggs

Freshly ground pepper to taste

DRESS IT UP Cholula or other hot sauce

1. Heat 1 tablespoon of the olive oil in a large cast-iron or nonstick skillet over medium-high heat. Add the sausage and cook, breaking up the meat with a wooden spoon, until no longer pink, about 5 minutes. Transfer to a large bowl, leaving any fat behind in the pan.

2. Add the damp kale to the pan. Cover and cook over medium-low heat for 5 minutes. Stir in ¼ teaspoon of the salt. If the kale seems very dry, add 2 tablespoons water. Continue to cook, covered, until the kale is mostly tender, 3 to 5 more minutes. Transfer to the bowl with the sausage.

3. Add the remaining 2 tablespoons olive oil to the pan and heat over medium heat. Add the frozen sweet potatoes, cover, and cook for 12 minutes, stirring once.

4. Return the sausage and kale to the pan, stirring to combine with the sweet potatoes. Make 4 indentations in the mixture and crack an egg into each. Cover the pan and cook until the eggs are set to your liking, 5 to 8 minutes. Sprinkle the eggs with the remaining ¼ teaspoon salt and pepper, and serve with the Cholula, if using.

SAUCY SIMMERED EGGS

MAKES 4 SERVINGS

A sprinkling of creamy feta gives this delicious dish briny, salty pop. If you prefer, skip the toast and serve this flavorful sauce over cooked rice or orzo.

2 tablespoons olive oil

1 cup chopped onion

¼ teaspoon plus ⅛ teaspoon kosher salt

¾ teaspoon Italian seasoning or dried oregano

2½ cups marinara sauce (20 ounces)

4 large eggs

2 ounces feta cheese, crumbled (½ cup)

4 large slices bread, toasted

DRESS IT UP Chopped dill and/or mint

1. Heat the olive oil in a large skillet over medium heat. Add the onion and ¼ teaspoon of the salt. Cook, stirring occasionally, until the onion is tender, about 5 minutes. Add the Italian seasoning and cook for another minute. Add the marinara sauce, bring to a simmer, and cook for about 3 minutes, stirring occasionally.

2. Make 4 indentations in the simmering sauce and crack an egg into each one. Sprinkle the feta around the eggs. Cover and cook over medium heat until the eggs are set to your liking, 5 to 8 minutes. Serve with the toast and chopped dill and/or mint, if desired.

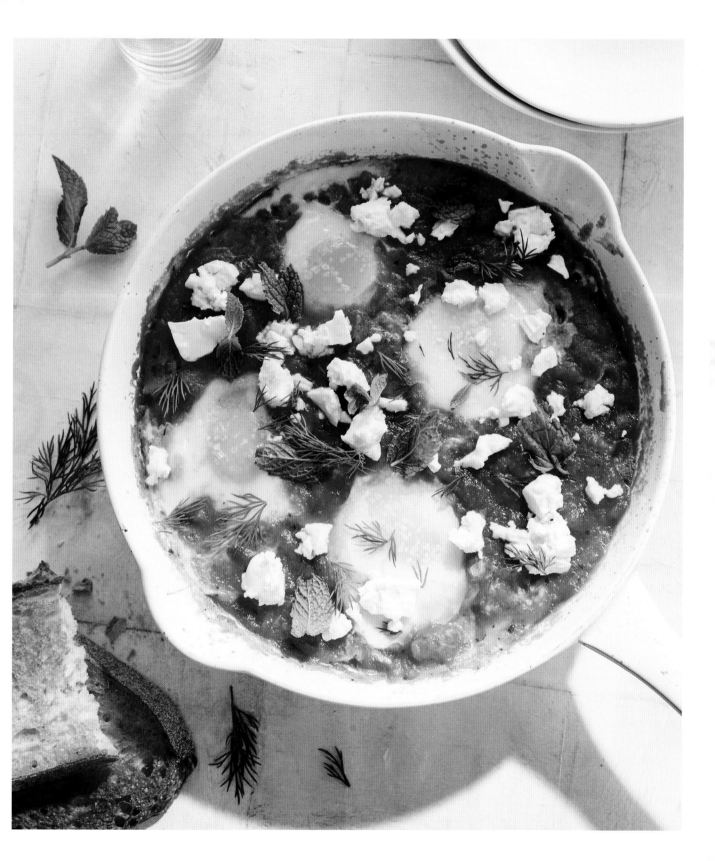

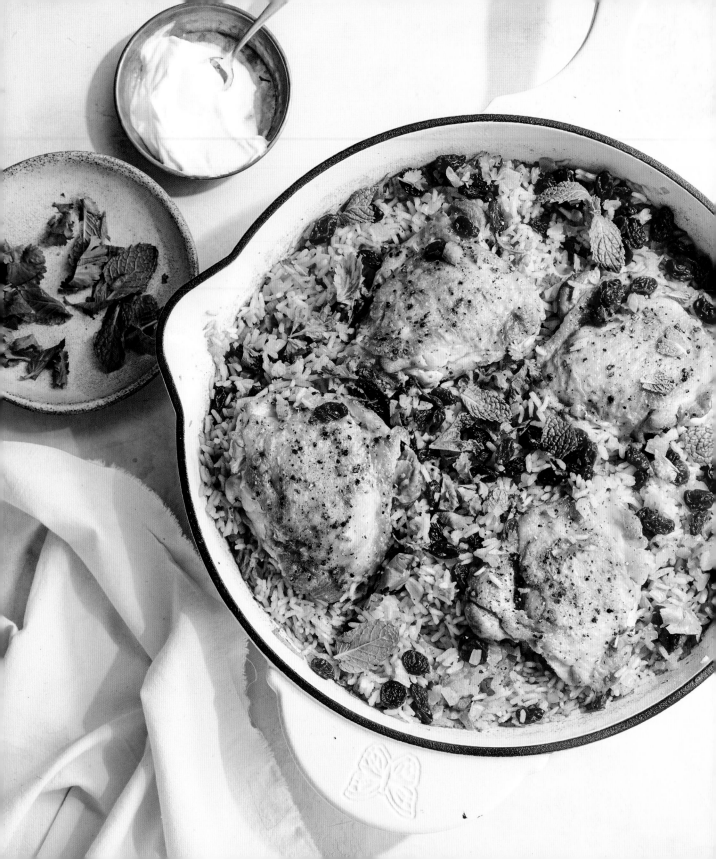

Spiced Chicken and Rice

MAKES 4 SERVINGS

I debated whether or not this was a "bare minimum dinner" when it comes to cleanup. Browning chicken thighs is not a quiet, clean task. There's a lot of spatter. But the convenience of cooking chicken and rice together in one pan won out—plus this dish is plain-old delicious! Use a spatter guard over the pan while the chicken cooks to minimize the mess.

4 bone-in, skin-on chicken thighs (about 1½ pounds)

1½ teaspoons kosher salt, divided

1 tablespoon coconut or canola oil

1 cup chopped yellow onion

2 teaspoons garam masala

½ teaspoon ground turmeric

1½ cups long-grain white rice

2¼ cups chicken broth

½ cup raisins

DRESS IT UP Plain whole-milk Greek yogurt, chopped cilantro and/or mint

1. Pat the chicken thighs dry with paper towels and sprinkle both sides with ¾ teaspoon of the salt.

2. Heat the coconut oil in a large skillet over medium-high heat. Add the chicken, skin side down. Cook, undisturbed, until deeply golden brown on the bottom, 8 to 10 minutes. Transfer the thighs to a plate, skin side up.

3. Reduce the heat to medium-low. Add the onion to the fat left in the pan and cook, stirring occasionally, until tender, about 5 minutes. Add the remaining ¾ teaspoon salt, garam masala, and turmeric. Cook, stirring, for 1 minute. Add the rice and cook, stirring frequently, until the grains start to become translucent, 1 to 2 minutes. Add the broth, increase the heat to high, and stir to scrape up any brown bits on the bottom of the pan. Once the broth is simmering, reduce the heat to medium-low and nestle the chicken thighs, skin side up, into the rice. Cover and cook for 25 minutes.

4. Remove the pan from the heat. Sprinkle the raisins into the pan. Cover again and let sit for 5 minutes. Serve with dollops of yogurt and chopped cilantro and/or mint, if desired.

ROUND IT OUT Any Green Leaf Salad (page 193) and/or Quick Cukes (page 218)

Any Onion Frittata

MAKES 4 SERVINGS

When I say any onion for this deeply savory dish, I mean it: red, yellow, Spanish, sweet, even shallots, scallions, or leeks. The onion powder kicks the flavor up a notch, but it isn't essential.

2 tablespoons olive oil

2 cups sliced onions

¾ teaspoon kosher salt, divided

7 large eggs

⅓ cup plain full-fat yogurt or whole milk

½ teaspoon onion powder (optional)

¼ cup grated Parmesan cheese (about 1 ounce)

1. Preheat the oven to 350°F.

2. Heat the oil in a 10-inch, oven-safe skillet over medium-high heat. Add the onions and ¼ teaspoon of the salt. Reduce the heat to medium-low and cook, stirring occasionally, until the onions are tender, about 7 minutes. (If using scallions, cook them for only about 2 minutes.)

3. In the meantime, whisk together the eggs, yogurt, remaining ½ teaspoon salt, and onion powder, if using, in a medium bowl.

4. Once the onions are cooked, pour the egg mixture into the pan. Cook for 3 minutes, then sprinkle the Parmesan cheese over the top. Transfer to the oven and bake until just set, 12 to 14 minutes. Let stand for at least 5 minutes before slicing and serving.

ROUND IT OUT Everyday Broccoli (page 197) or Peas with Walnuts and Parm (page 213)

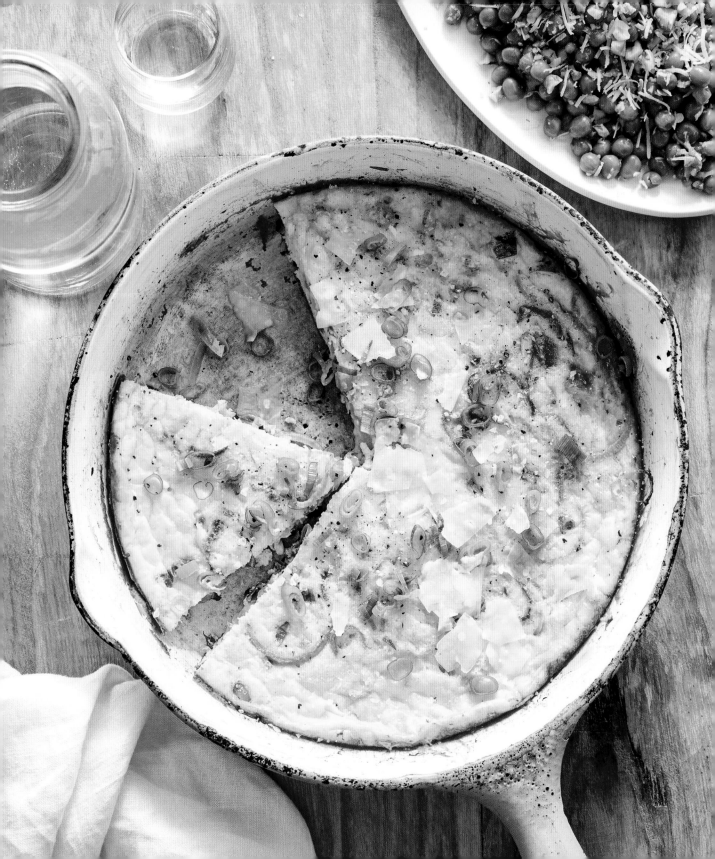

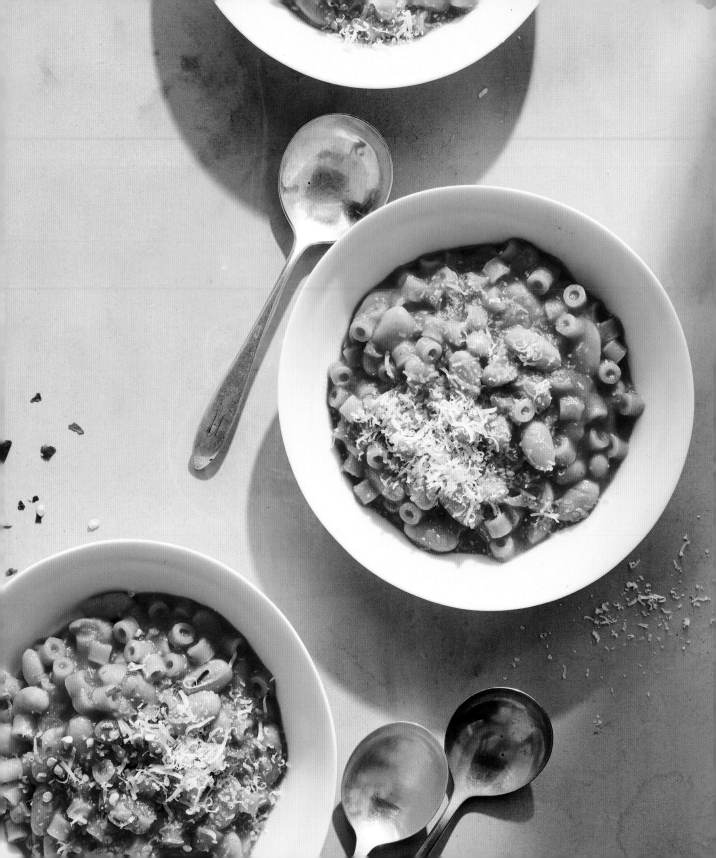

Magic White Bean and Tomato Stew

MAKES 4 SERVINGS

What's magic here, you ask? It's that such humble ingredients can come together into such a deeply flavored meal. This stew is also a beautiful example of how recipes are shared and adapted by a community of cooks. I first found a version of this Roman-inspired dish on Deb Perelman's blog, Smitten Kitchen. *Deb had in turn adapted it from food stylist and author Victoria Granof's book* Chickpeas. *As one does with recipes, I've subsequently made it my own, upping the portion sizes, changing the beans, and omitting the herb garnish. It's one of my all-time favorite bare minimum dinners.*

¼ cup olive oil, plus more for serving

4 cloves garlic, peeled and lightly smashed

1 6-ounce can tomato paste

2 15-ounce cans cannellini beans, rinsed and drained

1 cup ditalini or other small pasta

1½ teaspoons kosher salt

DRESS IT UP Crushed red pepper, grated Parmesan cheese

1. Heat the olive oil in a medium pot over medium heat. Add the garlic cloves and cook, stirring occasionally, until they are lightly golden, 2 to 3 minutes. Add the tomato paste and cook, stirring, for 1 minute. (Be careful, as it may spatter.)

2. Add 4 cups water, the cannellini beans, pasta, and salt. Bring to a boil, then reduce the heat to a simmer. Cook until the pasta is tender and much of the liquid is absorbed, about 15 minutes. Serve topped with a drizzle of olive oil. Dress it up with crushed red pepper and Parmesan cheese, if desired.

Skillet Pizza

MAKES 4 SERVINGS

If you have time, let the dough sit at room temperature for 30 minutes before cooking; it will be easier to stretch. If you don't have a cast-iron skillet, you can make this pizza on a baking sheet, although the crust won't be as crisp. If you have hot honey, use it here!

4 tablespoons olive oil, divided, plus more for drizzling

5 ounces shiitake mushrooms, sliced

½ teaspoon plus ⅛ teaspoon kosher salt, divided

2½ cups thinly sliced brussels sprouts (about 6 ounces)

1 pound white or whole-wheat pizza dough, thawed if frozen

1 cup whole-milk ricotta cheese, divided

Freshly ground black pepper to taste

¼ cup finely grated pecorino Romano or Parmesan cheese (about 1 ounce)

DRESS IT UP Honey or hot honey

1. Preheat the oven to 475°F.

2. Heat 2 tablespoons of the olive oil in a 12-inch cast-iron skillet over medium-high heat. Add the mushrooms and cook until they're golden and beginning to crisp, about 8 minutes. Stir in ¼ teaspoon of the salt, then transfer the mushrooms to a bowl.

3. Heat another 1 tablespoon olive oil in the skillet. Add the brussels sprouts and another ¼ teaspoon salt. Cook, stirring, until the sprouts begin to soften, about 4 minutes. Add ¼ cup water and continue to cook, stirring up any brown bits, until the sprouts are tender, about 2 more minutes. Transfer the sprouts to the bowl with the mushrooms and carefully wipe out the skillet.

4. Add the remaining 1 tablespoon olive oil to the skillet and heat over medium heat. Stretch the dough into a round and carefully place it

continued

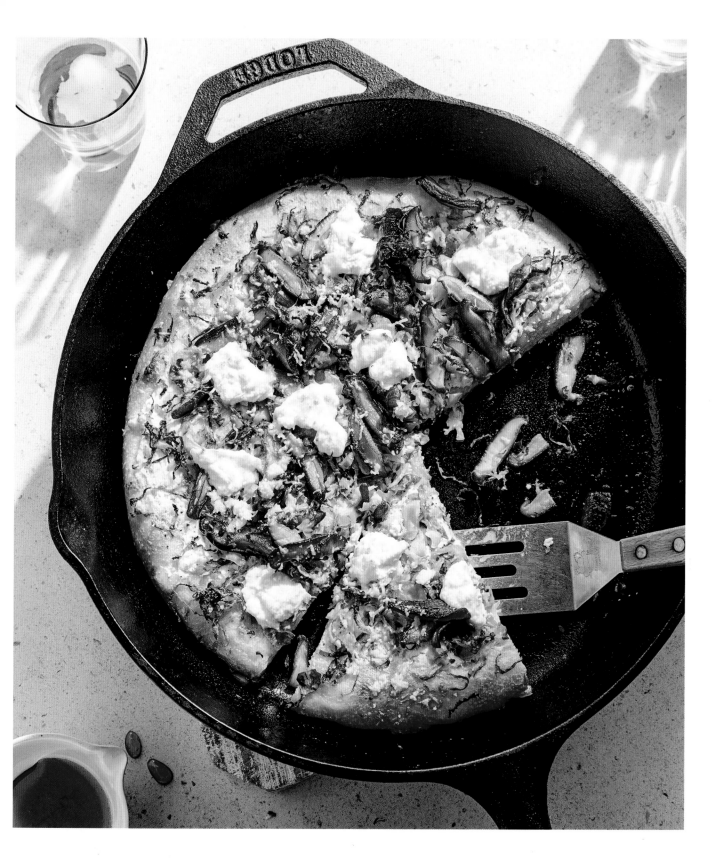

in the skillet, using a spoon to nudge it toward the edges if necessary. Spread ½ cup of the ricotta over the dough and season with the remaining ⅛ teaspoon salt and several grinds of pepper. Top evenly with the brussels sprouts and mushrooms, then dollop the remaining ½ cup ricotta over the vegetables. Scatter on the grated pecorino or Parm.

5. Transfer the skillet to the oven and bake until the crust is golden, 15 to 20 minutes. Let sit for 5 minutes, then slide the pizza onto a cutting board. Drizzle with more olive oil, slice, and serve, topped with honey or hot honey, if desired.

MAKE IT MEATY **Add sliced pepperoni and/or crumbled cooked Italian sausage before baking.**

Baked Chicken
with Artichokes and Feta

MAKES 4 SERVINGS

My friend Audrey shared this recipe with me. The secret, she says, is that the chicken bakes in the artichoke marinating liquid, giving your meal instant flavor. For a hit of saltiness she uses olives; I've swapped in feta cubes for a bit of creaminess in every bite. Use whichever you prefer and be sure to serve this over rice or with crusty bread to soak up all the flavorful juices in the baking dish.

4 boneless, skinless chicken breasts (about 1½ pounds)

½ teaspoon kosher salt, divided

Freshly ground black pepper to taste

1 12-ounce jar marinated artichoke hearts, undrained

4 ounces feta cheese, cut into ½-inch cubes

Olive oil, for drizzling

1. Preheat the oven to 375°F.

2. Season the undersides of the chicken breasts with ¼ teaspoon of the salt and lots of pepper. Place in a 13 × 9-inch baking dish, unseasoned sides up.

3. Pour the artichokes and the liquid in the jar over the chicken, then move the artichokes off the breasts. Nestle the feta into the artichokes. Sprinkle the chicken with the remaining ¼ teaspoon salt and more pepper. Drizzle the whole thing with olive oil. Bake until the chicken is cooked through (165°F on an instant-read thermometer), about 35 minutes.

ROUND IT OUT Crusty bread, rice, couscous, or Quinoa Pilaf (page 222)

BARE MINIMUM *Cleanup*

131

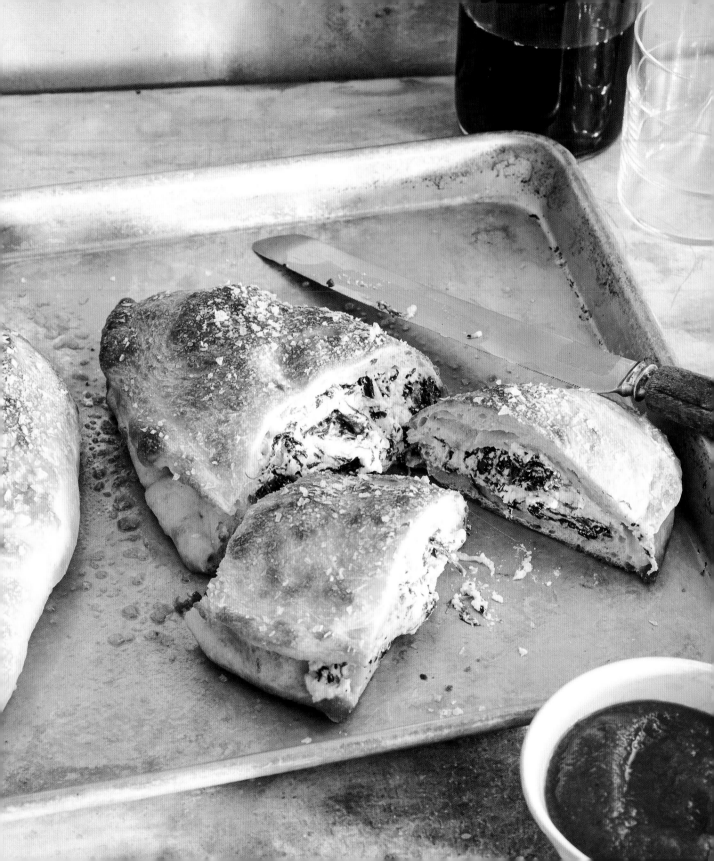

Spinach Calzones

MAKES 4 SERVINGS

Beyond pizza, this cheesy, comforting dinner is another great use for refrigerated or frozen dough, and it comes together in less time than it takes for delivery. As with the Skillet Pizza on page 128, if you let the dough stand at room temperature for a half hour before beginning the recipe, it will be easier to stretch and shape.

Olive oil, for greasing the pan and brushing the calzones

1 10-ounce package frozen chopped spinach, thawed and well drained

1½ cups whole-milk ricotta cheese

1 cup shredded low-moisture mozzarella cheese (about 4 ounces)

½ teaspoon kosher salt

¼ teaspoon crushed red pepper

1 pound white or whole-wheat pizza dough, thawed if frozen

Flaky sea salt to taste

Marinara sauce, for serving

1. Preheat the oven to 450°F. Grease a large rimmed baking sheet with olive oil.

2. In a large bowl, stir together the spinach, ricotta, mozzarella, kosher salt, and crushed red pepper.

3. Divide the dough into two equal parts. Stretch one dough ball into a flattish, round-ish shape. Spoon half of the spinach mixture on one half of the dough round. Fold the other half over the spinach mixture to make a half-moon. Pinch or fold the dough edges together to seal. Cut a small slit on top with a sharp knife. Repeat with the remaining dough and spinach mixture.

4. Transfer the calzones to the prepared baking sheet. Brush the tops with olive oil and sprinkle with flaky sea salt. Bake until the dough is cooked through and golden brown, 12 to 14 minutes. Let rest for 5 minutes, then cut each calzone in half and serve with marinara sauce.

MAKE IT MEATY Tuck in some pepperoni slices or cooked Italian sausage before you seal the calzones.

Three Ways with Chicken Soup

You can never have too many chicken soups in your repertoire.

CHICKEN AND "DUMPLING" SOUP

MAKES 4 TO 5 SERVINGS

Gnocchi may not be traditional soup dumplings, but they are little pillows of comforting deliciousness and my new favorite starchy add-in to chicken soup.

2 tablespoons olive oil

1 small yellow onion, chopped

2 carrots, peeled and chopped

2 celery stalks, chopped

½ teaspoon kosher salt

4 cups chicken broth (32 ounces)

1 pound refrigerated or shelf-stable gnocchi (such as De Cecco)

2 cups shredded cooked chicken (such as rotisserie)

1. Heat the olive oil in a large pot over medium heat. Add the onion, carrots, celery, and salt and cook, stirring occasionally, until just tender, about 5 minutes.

2. Add the broth and 1 cup water and bring to a boil. Add the gnocchi and cook until they float to the surface, 3 to 5 minutes (or according to the package directions). Stir in the chicken and serve.

CHICKEN TORTILLA SOUP

This recipe is also a delicious way to use up leftover Thanksgiving turkey.

2 tablespoons olive oil

1 cup chopped onion

2 celery stalks, chopped

½ teaspoon kosher salt, divided

1 teaspoon smoked paprika

4 cups chicken broth (32 ounces)

6 corn tortillas, torn or cut into 2 × 1-inch pieces

2 cups shredded cooked chicken (such as rotisserie) or turkey

1 cup roughly chopped cilantro

1. Heat the olive oil in a medium pot over medium heat. Add the onion, celery, and ¼ teaspoon of the salt. Cook, stirring occasionally, until the vegetables are tender, about 5 minutes. Add the smoked paprika and cook, stirring, for another minute.

2. Add the chicken broth and remaining ¼ teaspoon salt. Bring the soup to a boil over high heat, then stir in the tortilla pieces. Reduce the heat to medium-low, cover, and simmer for 15 minutes.

3. Stir in the chicken and cilantro and serve.

MISO CHICKEN RAMEN

MAKES 4 SERVINGS

Ginger and probiotic-rich miso enrich the broth in this super-fast and super-satisfying riff on ramen. There is a high proportion of noodles to broth here, because, well, noodles! Feel free to use two packages of instant ramen soup noodles; just discard the seasoning packets.

6 cups chicken broth (48 ounces)

1½ tablespoons finely chopped fresh ginger

1 tablespoon white miso paste

6 ounces dried ramen noodles

2 cups shredded cooked chicken (such as rotisserie)

4 cups torn spinach leaves or baby spinach (about 2 ounces)

DRESS IT UP Sliced scallions, sriracha or sambal oelek

1. In a medium pot, bring the chicken broth to a simmer over medium-high heat. Whisk in the ginger and miso. Simmer for about 5 minutes. Add the noodles and cook until al dente, about 3 minutes (or according to the package directions).

2. In the meantime, divide the chicken and spinach into 4 large bowls. Using tongs, portion the cooked noodles into the bowls. Ladle the broth over the top and serve with scallions and/or hot sauce, if desired.

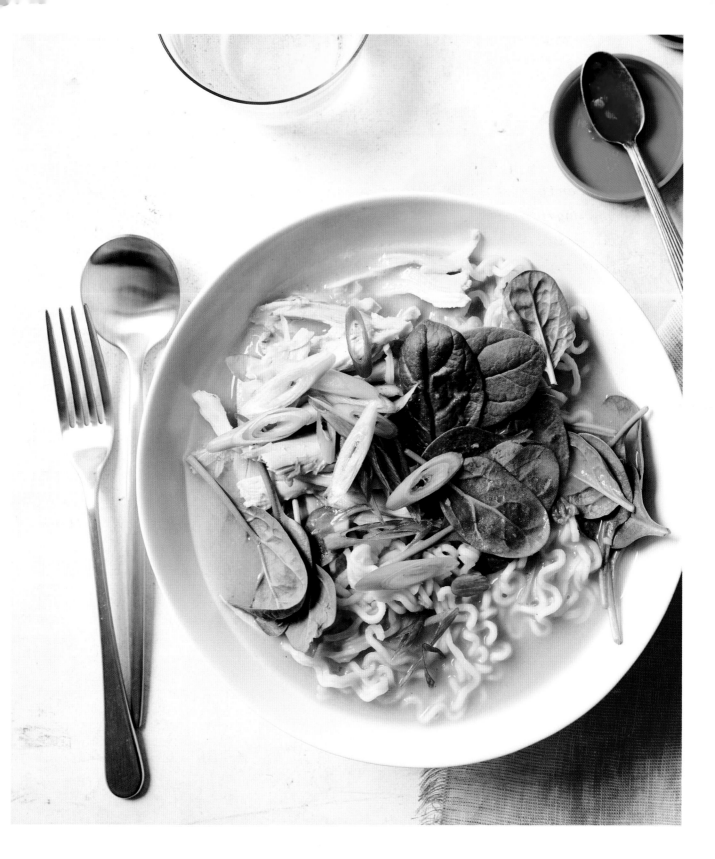

Layered Ravioli Bake

MAKES 4 TO 6 SERVINGS

Choose any ravioli filling you like for this easy, cheesy baked pasta. This plus a salad makes four servings in my always-hungry family, but if you're lighter eaters or serve it with multiple side dishes, you can probably stretch it to six.

Olive oil or nonstick cooking spray, for greasing the pan

3 cups marinara sauce (24 ounces)

2 9-ounce packages refrigerated ravioli

1 cup shredded low-moisture mozzarella cheese

¼ cup panko breadcrumbs

2 tablespoons grated Parmesan cheese

1. Preheat the oven to 400°F. Grease a broiler-safe 8 × 8-inch baking dish with olive oil or nonstick cooking spray.

2. Spread ½ cup of the sauce in the prepared dish. Add one package of ravioli in a mostly single layer. Add another 1½ cups sauce, the second package of ravioli, and then the remaining 1 cup sauce. Top with the mozzarella, panko, and Parmesan cheese.

3. Bake for 25 minutes. Heat the broiler and broil until the sauce is bubbly and the top is golden brown, 3 to 5 minutes.

Smoky Baked Potatoes

MAKES 4 SERVINGS

Smoked trout takes the place of the more traditional bacon in this classic easy dinner. The trout is unexpected, delicious, and even more low-effort since there's no cooking involved. If you're in a rush, feel free to microwave the potatoes. But, if you can, bake them in the oven for a delicious, crisp skin. In my opinion, it makes the meal.

4 large russet potatoes, well scrubbed

1 tablespoon olive oil

½ teaspoon kosher salt

Unsalted butter, softened, for serving

6 ounces smoked trout

2 scallions, trimmed and chopped, or ¼ cup chopped chives

DRESS IT UP Sour cream, flaky sea salt, freshly ground black pepper

1. Preheat the oven to 425°F. Line a rimmed baking sheet with parchment paper.

2. Prick the potatoes a few times with the tines of a fork, then rub them with the olive oil and sprinkle with the salt. Place on the prepared baking sheet and bake until very tender, 40 to 50 minutes (depending on the size), flipping them over after 30 minutes. Remove from the oven and let sit for 10 minutes.

3. Split the potatoes and top with the butter, trout, and scallions. Dress them up with sour cream, flaky sea salt, and pepper, if desired.

ROUND IT OUT Any Green Leaf Salad (page 193), Everyday Broccoli (page 197), or Asparagus with Garlicky Mayo (page 210)

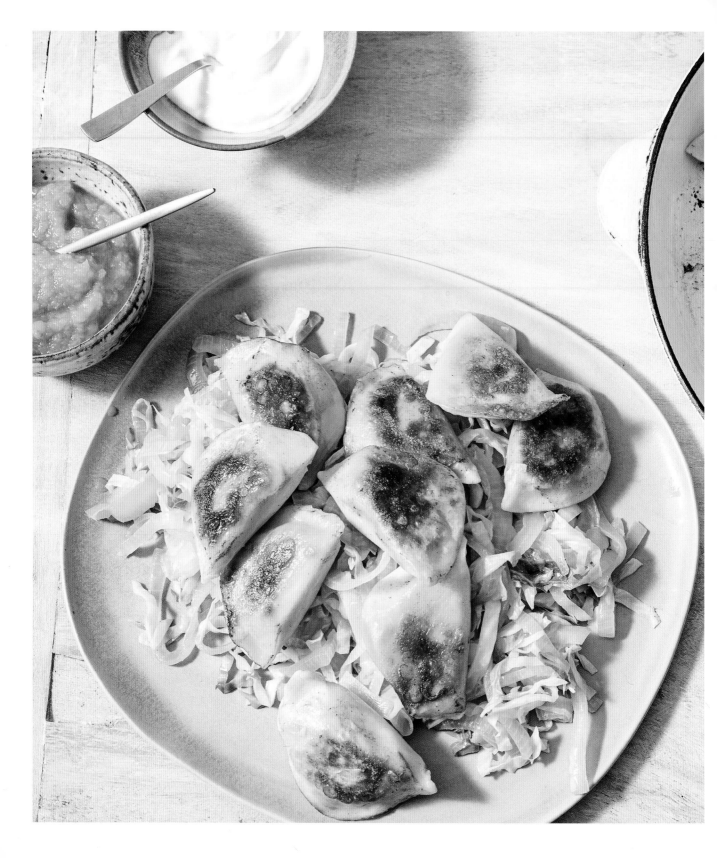

One-Pan Pierogi Supper

MAKES 4 SERVINGS

This is a pretty traditional way to serve Polish-style dumplings, and I love it, especially on an evening that calls for comfort food. This recipe uses a pound of refrigerated or frozen pierogi; choose your favorite filling. If that means opening two packages (not all packages are the same size), you can either make all of the pierogi and have leftovers, or you can freeze any extras and cook them later. Chances are, people will clamor for a repeat. Oh, and don't skip the sour cream and applesauce— they're essential.

2 tablespoons unsalted butter, divided

1 tablespoon olive oil

1 yellow onion, sliced

1 teaspoon kosher salt, divided

4 cups sliced green cabbage (about 12 ounces)

1 tablespoon apple cider vinegar

1 pound refrigerated or frozen pierogi

Sour cream and applesauce, for serving

1. Heat 1 tablespoon of the butter and the olive oil in a large skillet or sauté pan over medium heat. Add the onion and ¼ teaspoon of the salt. Reduce the heat to medium-low and cook until the onion is just tender, about 5 minutes. Add the cabbage and remaining ¾ teaspoon salt. Cook, tossing occasionally with tongs, until the cabbage is almost tender, about 7 minutes. Add the vinegar and toss again. Transfer to a serving plate.

2. Heat the remaining 1 tablespoon butter in the same pan over medium heat. Add the pierogi in a single layer of concentric circles. Add ¼ cup water, cover, and steam until the pierogi are tender and brown and crisp on the bottom, 5 to 7 minutes. Place on the serving plate over the cabbage mixture. Serve with sour cream and applesauce.

Za'atar Roast Chicken

MAKES 4 TO 6 SERVINGS

Za'atar is a spice blend with roots in the Middle East. It includes sesame seeds, oregano, and sumac, a bright, lemony spice. Get a head start on this dinner by putting the chicken in the yogurt mixture in the morning and letting it marinate in the refrigerator all day.

2 yellow onions, sliced

1 5-ounce container plain whole-milk Greek yogurt (about ⅔ cup)

3 tablespoons olive oil, divided, plus more for greasing the pan

2 tablespoons za'atar

2¼ teaspoons kosher salt, divided

1 chicken, cut into 8 pieces

1 pint cherry tomatoes

ROUND IT OUT Crusty bread, Any Green Leaf Salad (page 193), and/or Quinoa Pilaf (page 222)

1. Preheat the oven to 400°F. Lightly grease a rimmed baking sheet with olive oil.

2. Spread out the onions in a single layer on the prepared baking sheet.

3. In a large bowl, stir together the yogurt, 2 tablespoons of the olive oil, the za'atar, and 2 teaspoons of the kosher salt. Add the chicken pieces and turn to coat. Place the chicken, skin side up, on top of the onions on the baking sheet, leaving some space between each piece. Scrape out any of the remaining yogurt mixture in the bowl and spread it on the chicken. Roast for 30 minutes.

4. In a small bowl, toss the tomatoes with the remaining 1 tablespoon olive oil and remaining ¼ teaspoon salt. After the chicken has roasted for 30 minutes, add the tomatoes to the baking sheet and roast for an additional 30 minutes. Transfer the chicken to a platter. Use tongs to transfer the onions and tomatoes to a small bowl and serve them alongside the chicken.

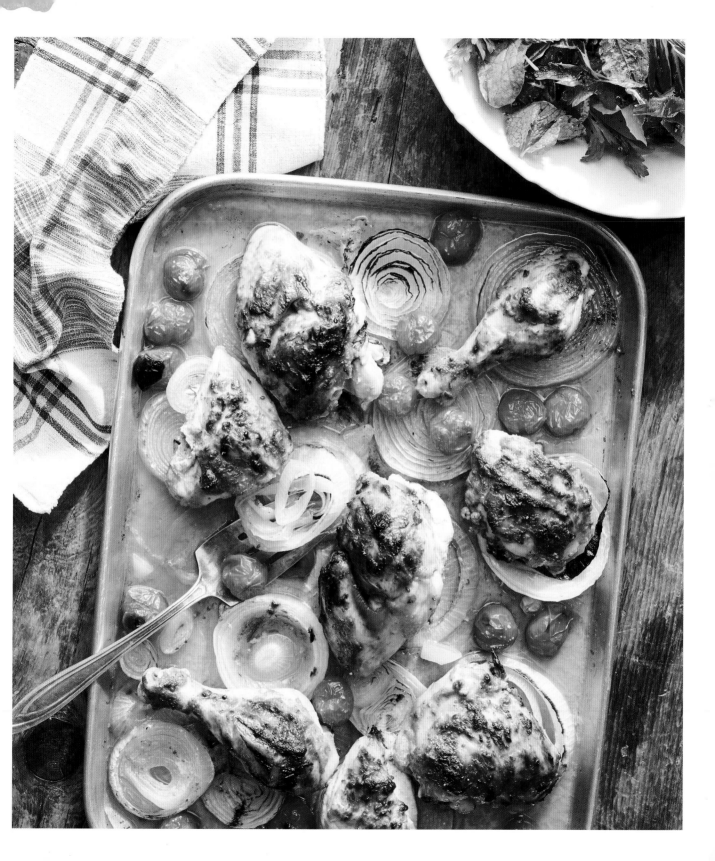

Roast Pork Loin with Fennel and Apples

MAKES 6 SERVINGS

This one-pan meal is dressy enough for a holiday but simple enough for a low-fuss Sunday supper. Plus, depending on the size of your crowd, it makes enough pork for sandwiches later in the week.

2½ pounds sweet potatoes, well scrubbed and cut into ½-inch-thick half-moons

2 Honeycrisp apples, cored and cut into wedges

1 fennel bulb, trimmed and cut into wedges and fronds chopped

3 tablespoons olive oil, divided

2 teaspoons kosher salt, divided

Freshly ground black pepper to taste

1 2½–3-pound pork loin

2 tablespoons Dijon mustard, plus more for serving

1. Preheat the oven to 400°F.

2. Combine the sweet potatoes, apples, and fennel wedges in a large roasting pan. Drizzle with 2 tablespoons of the olive oil and sprinkle with 1 teaspoon of the salt plus a few generous grinds of pepper. Spread evenly in the roasting pan, leaving room in the center for the pork.

3. Rub the pork loin all over with the Dijon mustard. Sprinkle with the remaining 1 teaspoon salt and more pepper. Place in the roasting pan and drizzle with the remaining 1 tablespoon olive oil. Roast until the temperature on an instant-read thermometer inserted in the center of the meat reaches 145°F, 55 to 60 minutes. Turn off the oven. Transfer the pork to a large cutting board and return the roasting pan to the oven to keep the vegetables warm. Let the pork rest for 10 minutes.

4. Slice the pork and serve with the vegetable mixture. Garnish with the fennel fronds and serve with more Dijon, if desired.

One-Pot Bacon and Zucchini Pasta

MAKES 4 SERVINGS

Cooking pasta and sauce together in one pot seems like a miracle. The pasta absorbs most of the liquid, becoming tender and flavorful—no colander required. You'll end up with a little bit of saucy cooking liquid, which I like to serve with the pasta, and I confess that once I've eaten all of the meal, I tip the bowl to my mouth and slurp up the rest of that brothy goodness.

6 slices bacon

12 ounces penne pasta

2 small zucchini (or 1 medium), sliced into ½-inch-thick half-moons

1 pint cherry tomatoes, halved

1 red onion, sliced

1 teaspoon kosher salt

4 cups chicken broth (32 ounces)

Olive oil, for drizzling

DRESS IT UP Torn basil leaves, grated Parmesan cheese, crushed red pepper, flaky sea salt

1. Heat a large pot or Dutch oven over medium heat. Add the bacon and cook until crisp, about 3 minutes per side. Transfer to a paper towel–lined plate and discard the fat in the pan.

2. Add the pasta, zucchini, tomatoes, onion, and salt to the same pot. Add the broth and ½ cup water, or just enough to cover all of the ingredients. Bring the liquid to a boil and cook over medium-high heat, stirring occasionally to keep from sticking, until the pasta is tender and the liquid is greatly reduced, 9–11 minutes (after the liquid comes to a boil).

3. Divide the pasta mixture and broth among 4 shallow bowls, drizzle with olive oil, and crumble the bacon over the top. Dress it up with some basil, Parm, crushed red pepper, and/or sea salt, if desired.

V MAKE IT MEATLESS Skip the bacon altogether and use vegetable broth. Or for a meal that vegetarians and omnivores can share, cook the bacon (1 or 2 slices per person) in a second pan and crumble only over the meat eaters' portions.

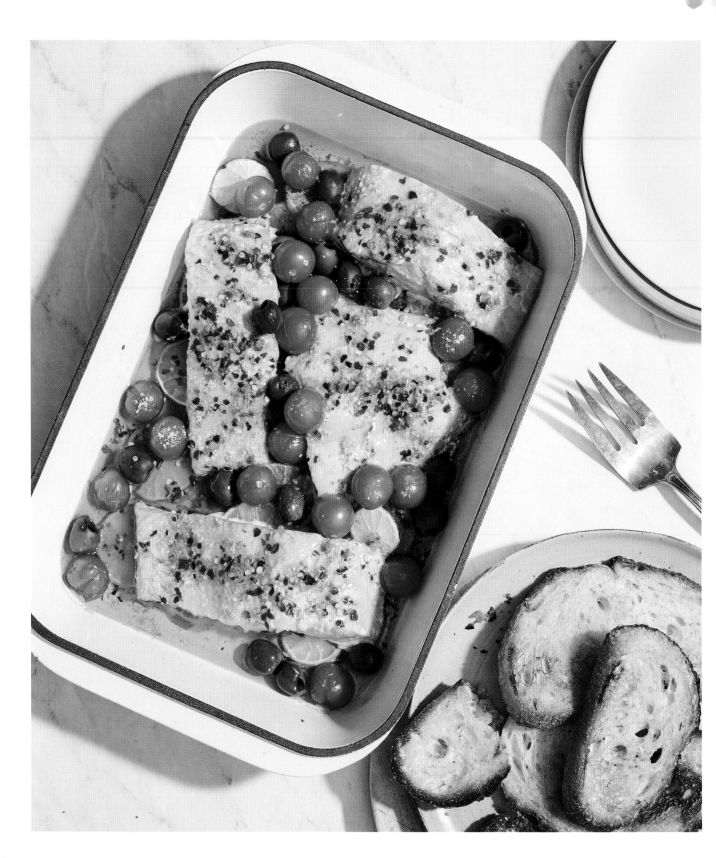

Chile-Lime Salmon

MAKES 4 SERVINGS

Roasting salmon low and slow is a game-changer for foolproof silky, tender fish. And, since this is salmon—not a pork shoulder—"slow" means about 20 minutes. Serve this with crusty bread for soaking up the chile-lime oil.

½ cup olive oil

2 limes

1 teaspoon crushed red pepper

1 teaspoon kosher salt, divided

4 5–6-ounce salmon fillets

1 cup cherry tomatoes

½ cup pitted olives (such as Castelvetrano)

Flaky sea salt to taste

1. Preheat the oven to 300°F.

2. Pour the olive oil into a small bowl. Zest the limes into the oil, then whisk in the crushed red pepper and ¼ teaspoon of the salt. Thinly slice the zested limes.

3. Spread out the lime slices in a 13 × 9-inch baking dish. Top with the salmon fillets. Sprinkle the salmon with the remaining ¾ teaspoon salt. Nestle the tomatoes and olives around the fish, and pour the olive oil mixture over it all.

4. Bake until the salmon is cooked to the level of doneness you prefer, 20 to 25 minutes for medium. Sprinkle flaky sea salt over everything and serve.

ROUND IT OUT Crusty bread, Quinoa Pilaf (page 222), and/or Everyday Broccoli (page 197)

Gnocchi Sheet Pan Supper

MAKES 4 SERVINGS

My mind was just a little bit blown when I discovered that gnocchi didn't need to be boiled, but instead could be roasted in the oven with veggies or sausage. And if that weren't reason enough to make this dish, this recipe is also an excellent way to use up any lingering sprigs of hardy herbs in your crisper.

1 pound refrigerated or shelf-stable gnocchi (such as De Cecco)

10 ounces button or cremini mushrooms, trimmed and quartered

3-5 sprigs woodsy herbs (such as rosemary, oregano, thyme, or sage; optional)

2 tablespoons olive oil, plus more for drizzling

½ teaspoon kosher salt

6 cups baby arugula

½ cup full-fat ricotta cheese

½ lemon

1. Preheat the oven to 425°F. Line a rimmed baking sheet with parchment paper.

2. Combine the gnocchi, mushrooms, and herbs, if using, on the prepared baking sheet. Add the olive oil and salt and toss to coat, then spread out the gnocchi and mushrooms in a single layer. Roast until the gnocchi are tender and the mushrooms are golden, about 20 minutes.

3. Divide the arugula into 4 shallow bowls or plates. Top with the gnocchi mixture, then dollop with the ricotta. Squeeze the lemon over the plates, drizzle with more olive oil, and serve.

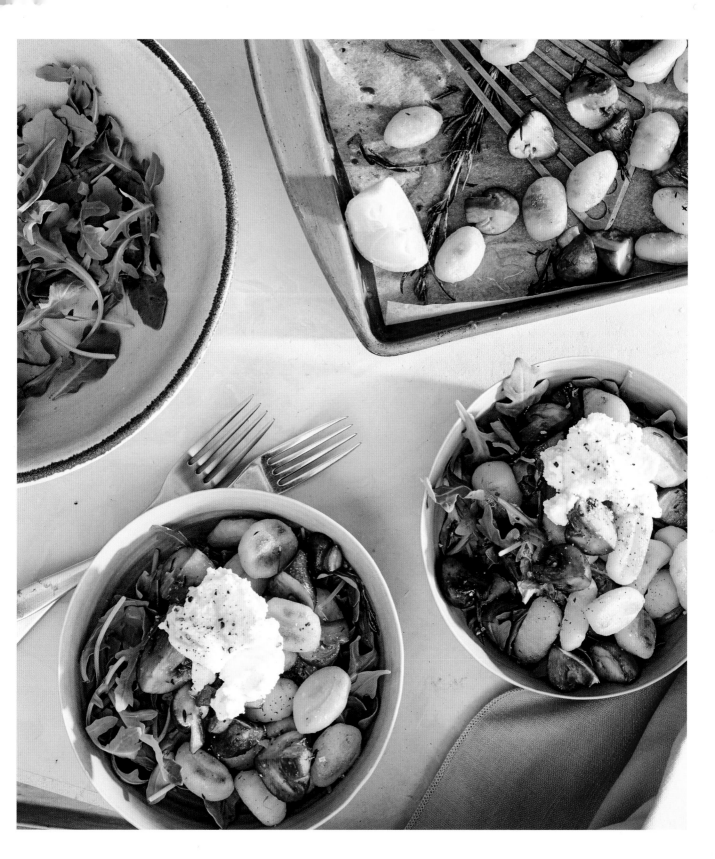

Greek Chicken Salad

Mayo combined with feta makes for a savory, satisfying dressing.

½ cup mayonnaise

4 ounces feta cheese, crumbled (about 1 cup)

2 tablespoons red wine vinegar

Freshly ground black pepper to taste

4 cups shredded cooked chicken (such as rotisserie)

½ cup pitted Kalamata or mixed Greek olives, chopped

¼ cup finely chopped red onion

1 pint cherry tomatoes, halved

2 mini (Persian) cucumbers, thinly sliced

Pita bread or pita chips, for serving

DRESS IT UP Chopped dill

In a large bowl, stir together the mayonnaise, feta, vinegar, and plenty of pepper, mashing the feta with the back of a spoon. Stir in the chicken, olives, red onion, and dill, if using. Serve with the tomatoes, cucumbers, and pita.

Mixed Grill

In this recipe, your "one pot" is your backyard grill or, in a pinch, indoor grill pan. This is one of my favorite summer meals, especially when we have people over, because it's so easy to double and so free-form. Good add-ons include sliced eggplant and halloumi, a delicious, salty cheese that actually stays intact on the grill. This mixed grill is also excellent for a mixed group of vegetarians and meat eaters since both sausages and tofu are involved. If you're only vegetarians, skip the sausage and double the tofu or add on halloumi.

1 14-ounce package extra-firm tofu

⅓ cup olive oil, plus more for drizzling and grilling

Grated zest and juice of 1 lemon

2 teaspoons ground coriander

1 teaspoon kosher salt, plus more for seasoning

1 teaspoon crushed red pepper

3 bell peppers, any color but green

3 medium zucchini

1 pound sweet or hot Italian sausages

2–4 pita bread rounds (depending on their size and your appetite)

DRESS IT UP Chopped mint, parsley, basil, and/or cilantro, flaky sea salt, plain whole-milk Greek yogurt

1. Place the tofu on a paper towel–lined plate. Top with another paper towel and another plate. Place a box of broth or a can of tomatoes on the top plate to weight it down. Let the tofu drain for about 10 minutes.

2. Meanwhile, whisk together the olive oil, lemon zest and juice, coriander, salt, and crushed red pepper in a 2-cup liquid measuring cup.

3. Cut the bell peppers into 4 or 5 wide chunks each, discarding the core and seeds. Trim the zucchini and slice them into long, thin planks. Put the peppers and zucchini in a large, shallow dish. Drizzle with plenty of olive oil and season with salt, then toss to make sure everything is well coated.

continued

BARE MINIMUM *Cleanup*

4. Slice the tofu lengthwise into 4 slabs and place them on a plate. Drizzle the tofu with olive oil and season with salt.

5. Preheat the grill to medium-high. Grease well with olive oil. Grill the vegetables and tofu until they are tender and browned and grill marks have appeared, 4 to 5 minutes. Transfer the vegetables and tofu to the same baking dish and pour the lemon-coriander oil over. Use tongs to move things around to make sure everything is well coated. Top with chopped herbs, if using.

6. Grill the sausages, turning occasionally, until cooked through, about 10 minutes. Add the pita to the grill for the final minute. Serve with the cooked vegetables and tofu, along with flaky sea salt and yogurt for dolloping, if desired.

One-Pan Chicken Dinner

MAKES 4 SERVINGS

This is a bare minimum dinner that feels like an event. Since you're preheating the skillet, you can cook the chicken directly in the pan, no roasting rack required. Don't skip squeezing the lemon over the entire dish. The acid perks everything up.

1 4-pound chicken, gizzards removed

2 teaspoons kosher salt

Freshly ground black pepper

1 tablespoon olive oil

1½ pounds baby potatoes

1 lemon, halved

DRESS IT UP Flaky sea salt, chopped parsley or tarragon, Dijon mustard

1. Preheat the oven to 450°F. Place a 12-inch or larger cast-iron skillet in the oven as it heats.

2. Pat the chicken dry with paper towels. Sprinkle a little less than half of the kosher salt on its underside. Sprinkle the rest of the salt on top of the chicken, along with plenty of pepper.

3. Once the oven is preheated, carefully remove the skillet. Place the chicken breast-side up in the skillet; you should hear a sizzle. Drizzle with the olive oil and roast for 30 minutes.

4. Carefully remove the skillet from the oven. Reduce the oven temperature to 375°F. Add the potatoes to the pan with the chicken. They will be mounded up in places, and that's fine. Nestle in the lemon halves. Continue to roast until an instant-read thermometer inserted into the meatiest part of the thigh reaches 165°F, 35 to 45 minutes. Transfer the chicken

continued

and lemons to a cutting board. Spread the potatoes into a single layer in the skillet and return them to the oven. Continue roasting the potatoes for 15 minutes while the chicken rests.

5. Carve the chicken and place on a serving platter. Transfer the potatoes to a serving bowl. Squeeze the lemon halves over the chicken and potatoes. Sprinkle the potatoes with flaky sea salt, top with herbs, and serve with Dijon mustard for dabbing, if desired.

ROUND IT OUT Any Green Leaf Salad (page 193), Eat-with-Everything Slaw (page 196), or Caprese-ish Salad (page 221)

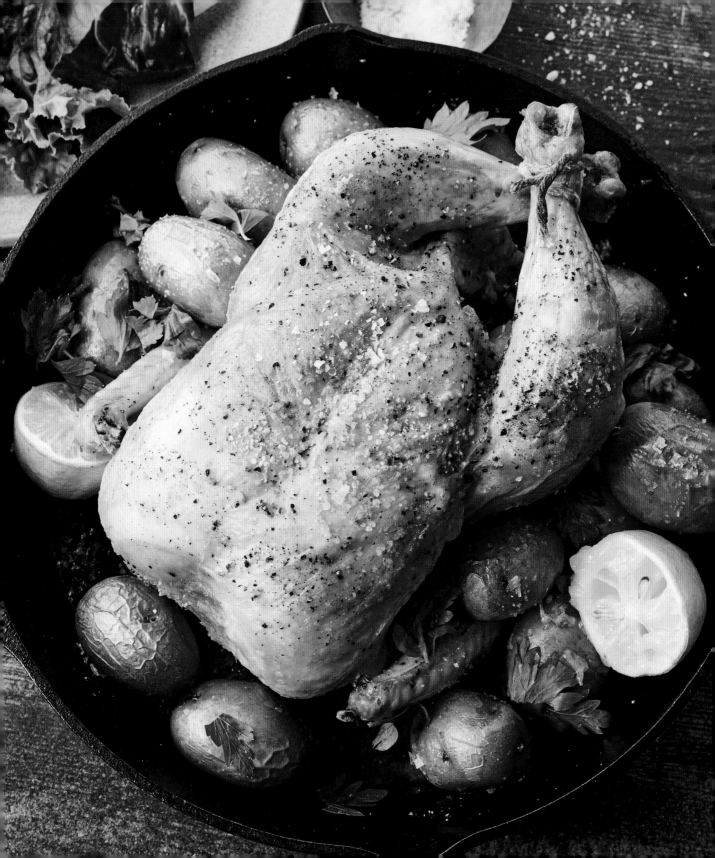

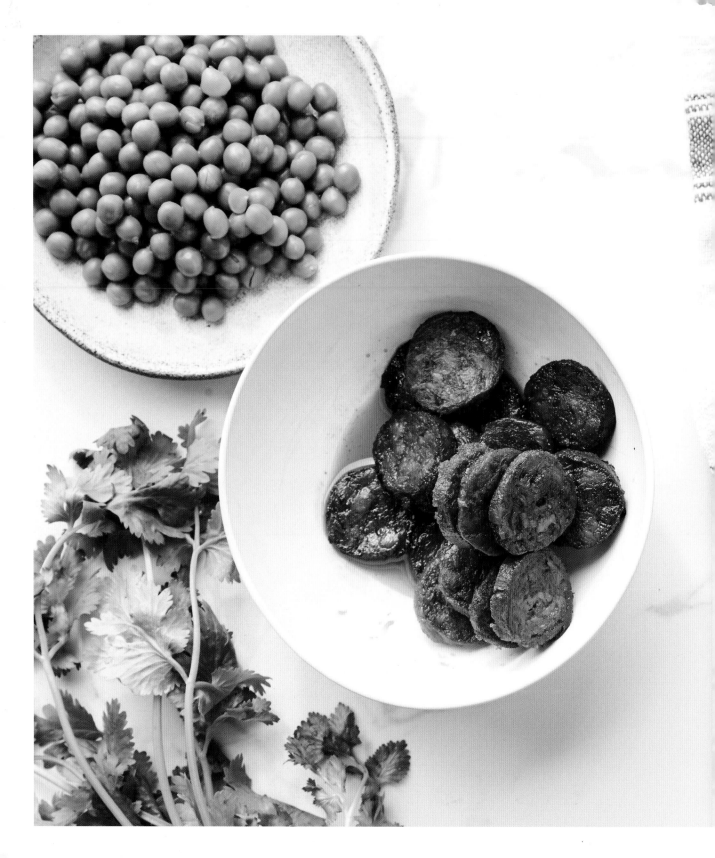

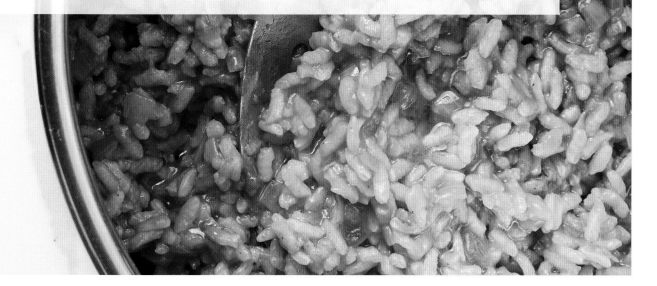

BARE MINIMUM
Hands-On Time

Recipes for the Instant Pot
or Slow Cooker

Instant Pot Bean with Bacon Soup

MAKES 4 TO 6 SERVINGS

Growing up, Campbell's Bean with Bacon was my favorite soup, even though there was no detectable bacon in the broth. I wanted to recreate that flavor in my Instant Pot, but with actual bacon pieces and even some greens, because I can't help myself.

4 slices bacon

1 tablespoon tomato paste

4 cups chicken broth (32 ounces)

2 cups dried pinto beans or any similar-sized beans

1 teaspoon kosher salt

8 cups chopped escarole (about 1 large bunch)

Instant Pot Cooking Tip

Instant Pot timings are not an exact science. (Really, *no* recipe timings are an exact science.) If you open the pot and find that, say, your beans aren't tender, or your meat is still a little tough, simply relock the lid and cook for 5 to 10 more minutes. It may take a few minutes for you to be able to reseal the pot since the contents are so hot. Once you do lock the lid and start the cook time again, the pot will come up to pressure much faster than before since the ingredients inside the pot are already very hot.

1. Set the Instant Pot or other multicooker to Sauté. Using kitchen shears, cut the bacon into 1-inch pieces directly into the pot. Cook, stirring frequently, until browned and crisped, about 5 minutes. Press Cancel and use a slotted spoon to transfer the bacon to a paper towel–lined plate.

2. Set the Instant Pot to Sauté again. Add the tomato paste and stir until fragrant and incorporated into the bacon fat, about 1 minute. Add the chicken broth and 2 cups water. Stir, scraping up any brown bits on the bottom of the pot with a wooden spoon. Add the beans and salt. Press Cancel. Lock the lid and set to cook on high pressure for 35 to 40 minutes (longer if your beans are on the older side).

3. When cooking is complete, press Cancel and let the pressure release naturally for 10 minutes. Carefully quick-release the remaining pressure and remove the lid. Stir in the escarole until wilted, then serve.

Instant Pot Lemony Shrimp Risotto

MAKES 4 SERVINGS

I am always amazed when I make risotto in the pressure cooker. It comes out perfectly every time. I like the flavor of chicken broth here, but use veggie if you prefer.

3 tablespoons olive oil, divided

1 pound raw large shrimp (16–20 per pound), peeled and deveined

1 teaspoon kosher salt, divided

Grated zest of 1 lemon

⅛ teaspoon crushed red pepper (optional)

¼ cup chopped shallot

1½ cups Arborio rice

4 cups chicken or vegetable broth (32 ounces)

4 cups torn spinach leaves or baby spinach (about 2 ounces)

1 tablespoon unsalted butter

1. Set the Instant Pot or other multicooker to Sauté and add 1 tablespoon of the olive oil. When the oil is hot, add the shrimp and ¼ teaspoon of the salt. Sauté the shrimp until just cooked through, 3 to 4 minutes, then transfer to a medium bowl. Press Cancel. Toss the shrimp with the lemon zest and crushed red pepper, if using.

2. Set the Instant Pot to Sauté again. Add the remaining 2 tablespoons olive oil and shallot and cook, stirring frequently, until the shallot begins to soften, 2 to 3 minutes. Add the rice and cook, stirring, until the rice is translucent, about 2 minutes. Add the broth and another ½ teaspoon salt. Stir to scrape up any brown bits on the bottom of the pot. Lock the lid and set to cook on high pressure for 6 minutes.

3. When cooking is complete, press Cancel and carefully quick-release the pressure.

4. Stir for a minute or two to thicken the risotto, then add the spinach, butter, and remaining ¼ teaspoon salt, stirring just until the spinach is wilted. Serve topped with the shrimp and their juices.

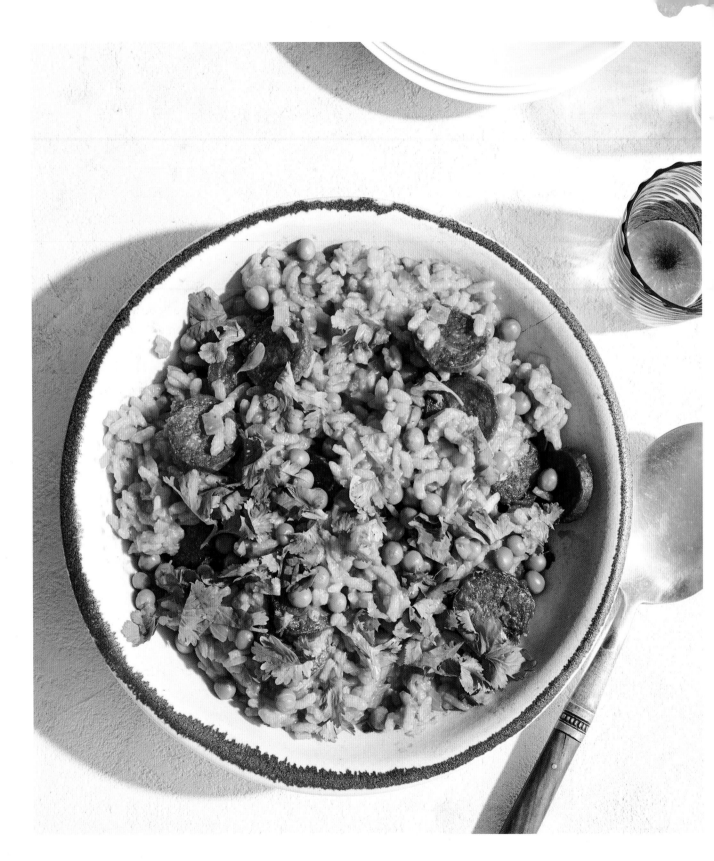

Instant Pot "Pae-sotto"

As the name suggests, this hearty meal is a mash-up of Spanish paella and Italian risotto. Like everything that comes out of the Instant Pot, this dish is super-hot! Let it sit for about 5 minutes to cool slightly and thicken up before serving.

1 tablespoon olive oil

8 ounces Spanish chorizo, sliced ¼ inch thick

1 cup chopped onion

1¼ teaspoons kosher salt, divided

1 teaspoon smoked paprika

1½ cups Arborio rice

2 tablespoons tomato paste

4 cups vegetable broth (32 ounces)

1 cup frozen peas

2 teaspoons lemon juice

DRESS IT UP Chopped cilantro

V MAKE IT MEATLESS Skip the chorizo and start with 2 tablespoons olive oil. If you're cooking for both vegetarians and omnivores, cook the chorizo in a skillet on the stove-top and add it only to the meat eaters' portions.

1. Set the Instant Pot or other multicooker to Sauté and add the olive oil. When the oil is hot, add the chorizo. Sauté until the chorizo renders its fat and begins to get crisp, 2 to 3 minutes. Transfer the chorizo to a bowl, leaving the fat in the pot.

2. Add the onion and ¼ teaspoon of the salt. Sauté, stirring frequently, until the onion begins to soften, about 3 minutes. Add the smoked paprika and cook, stirring, for 1 minute. Add the rice and cook, stirring, until the rice is translucent, about 2 minutes. Add the tomato paste and cook, stirring, for another minute. Add the broth and the remaining 1 teaspoon salt. Stir to scrape up any brown bits on the bottom of the pot. Lock the lid and set to cook on high pressure for 6 minutes.

3. When cooking is complete, press Cancel and carefully quick-release the pressure.

4. Stir for a minute or two to thicken the risotto. Then stir in the peas, lemon juice, chorizo, and cilantro, if using.

Instant Pot Chickpea, Kale, and Sausage Stew

MAKES 6 SERVINGS

Just five ingredients and some water give you a healthy, big-flavor stew. The chickpeas are the heart of this earthy meal. Cooking them from dried, instead of using canned, adds extra oomph to the broth.

1 tablespoon olive oil, plus more for drizzling

8 ounces sweet or hot Italian pork sausage, removed from its casings

1 cup dried chickpeas

1½ teaspoons kosher salt

1 bunch lacinato kale, stems removed and leaves torn into bite-sized pieces (about 6 cups)

1. Set the Instant Pot or other multicooker to Sauté and add the olive oil. When the oil is hot, add the sausage and cook, breaking up the meat with a wooden spoon, until no longer pink, about 5 minutes. Press Cancel and transfer the sausage to a bowl.

2. Add 6 cups water to the pot and stir with the wooden spoon to scrape up any brown bits on the bottom. Add the chickpeas and salt. Lock the lid and set to cook on high pressure for 35 to 40 minutes (longer if your beans are larger or on the older side).

3. When cooking is complete, press Cancel and carefully quick-release the pressure. Remove the lid and stir in the kale. Set the lid on the pot but don't lock it, and let the kale wilt for 5 minutes. Add the sausage back to the pot. Stir and serve, drizzled with more olive oil.

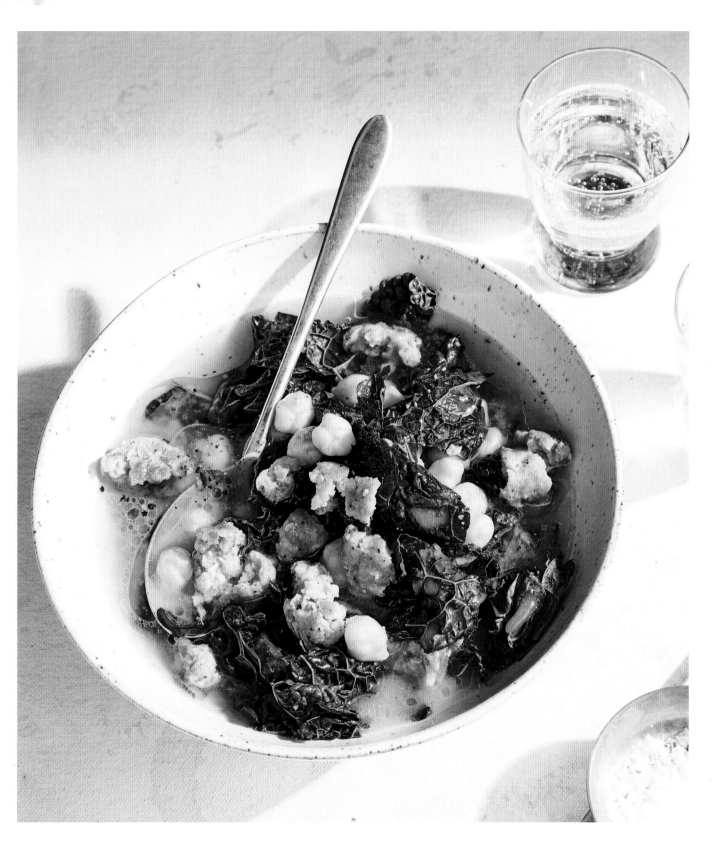

Instant Pot Smoky Beef Chili

MAKES 8 SERVINGS

Most stew and chili recipes for the Instant Pot ask you to sear the meat in batches, making sure each side is well browned. That method imparts tons of flavor, but if you have other big-flavored ingredients, as in this stew, you can cut a few corners. You'll save time and still have a deeply satisfying dish.

2 tablespoons canola or other neutral oil

1 medium onion, chopped

2 teaspoons ground cumin

2 teaspoons kosher salt, divided

2 pounds beef stew meat cubes

1 chipotle chile in adobo sauce, chopped

1 28-ounce can diced tomatoes, with their juice

1½ pounds sweet potatoes, peeled and chopped

1 15-ounce can pinto beans, rinsed and drained

¼ cup chopped cilantro

1. Set the Instant Pot or other multicooker to Sauté and add the oil. When the oil is hot, add the onion and cook, stirring frequently, until softened, about 3 minutes. Add the cumin and 1 teaspoon of the salt and cook for 1 minute.

2. Add the beef and another ½ teaspoon salt. Let the beef brown, stirring once or twice, for 5 minutes. Stir in the chile, tomatoes, and 1 cup water, scraping up any brown bits on the bot-

tom of the pot. Lock the lid and set to cook on high pressure for 40 minutes.

3. When cooking is complete, press Cancel and let the pressure release naturally for 15 minutes. Carefully quick-release the remaining pressure and remove the lid. Stir in the sweet potatoes, beans, and remaining ½ teaspoon salt. Lock the lid and set to cook on high pressure for 5 minutes. (You may need to wait a few minutes for the contents of the pot to cool before you can lock the lid again. The ingredients will come up to pressure much faster now than at the beginning of the recipe.)

4. When cooking is complete, press Cancel and carefully quick-release the pressure. Stir in the cilantro and serve.

Instant Pot Split-Pea Coconut Soup

MAKES 4 TO 6 SERVINGS

Inspired by the dal that I often order in Indian restaurants, this is a warmly spiced, creamy, and incredibly comforting soup. Serve it with naan, pita, or crusty bread to soak up every flavorful bite.

2 tablespoons coconut oil

1 cup chopped onion

2 carrots, peeled and finely chopped

1 tablespoon curry powder

½ teaspoon ground ginger

4 cups vegetable broth (32 ounces)

1½ cups yellow split peas, rinsed

2 teaspoons kosher salt

1 13.5-ounce can coconut milk (well shaken)

Juice of 1 lime

1. Set the Instant Pot or other multicooker to Sauté and add the coconut oil. When the oil is hot, add the onion and carrots and cook until tender, about 5 minutes. Stir in the curry powder and ginger and cook for 1 minute. Press Cancel.

2. Stir in the broth, split peas, and salt. Lock the lid and set to cook on high pressure for 15 minutes.

3. When cooking is complete, press Cancel and let the pressure release naturally for 10 minutes. Carefully quick-release the remaining pressure and remove the lid. Stir in the coconut milk and lime juice and serve.

ROUND IT OUT Naan, pita, or crusty bread

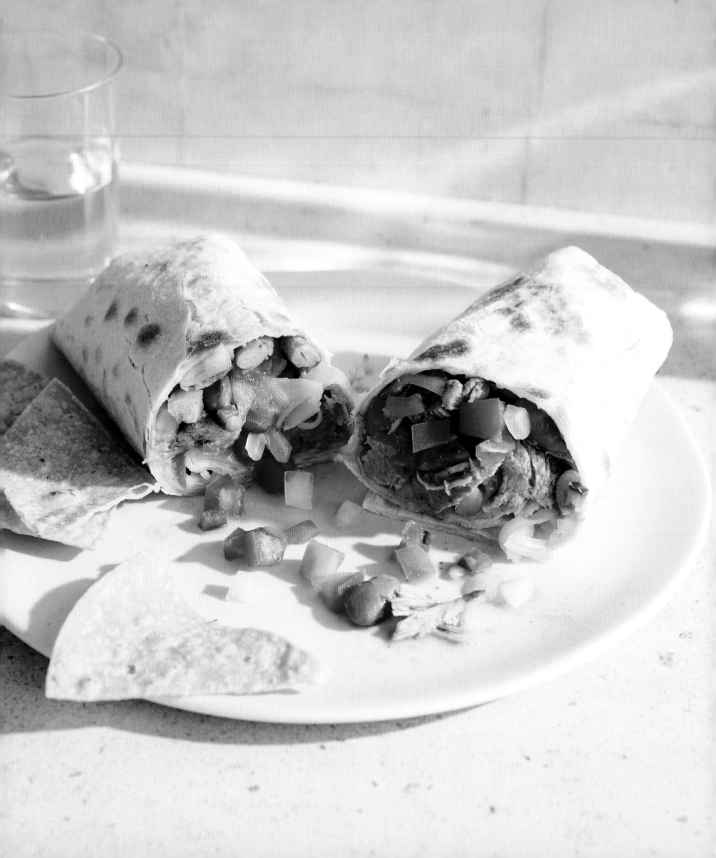

Instant Pot Pork and Bean Burritos

MAKES ENOUGH FILLING FOR 6 TO 8 BURRITOS

This recipe makes enough filling for about eight burritos. If you're serving only four people, freeze the remaining filling to assemble more burritos down the road. Or, for an even easier future dinner, assemble three or four additional burritos (be sure to increase the amount of cheese and salsa called for in the ingredient list) and freeze them in aluminum foil. To defrost, remove the foil and wrap in a paper towel. Microwave until heated through, 4 to 5 minutes, flipping after 2 minutes.

1 tablespoon ground cumin

1 teaspoon chili powder

3 teaspoons kosher salt, divided

2 pounds pork stew meat cubes

1 tablespoon canola or other neutral oil

1 cup dried pinto or cranberry beans

1 chipotle chile in adobo sauce, chopped

4 large flour tortillas, warmed

½ cup shredded cheddar cheese (about 2 ounces)

¼ cup salsa, or more if desired

1. In a large bowl, stir together the cumin, chili powder, and 2 teaspoons of the salt. Add the pork and toss to coat.

2. Set the Instant Pot or other multicooker to Sauté and add the oil. When the oil is hot, add the pork and brown, stirring once or twice, for 5 minutes. Press Cancel.

3. Add 3 cups water to the pot and use a wooden spoon to scrape up any brown bits. Add the beans, chipotle chile, and remaining 1 teaspoon salt. Lock the lid and set to cook on high pressure for 50 minutes.

4. When cooking is complete, press Cancel and let the pressure release naturally for 25 minutes.

5. Using a slotted spoon, add about 1 cup of the pork and bean mixture to the center of each warm tortilla. Top with shredded cheese and salsa. Roll up the burritos and serve.

Instant Pot Meatballs in Marinara

MAKES 4 SERVINGS

You can eat these tender, full-flavored, saucy meatballs as is—or tuck them into rolls for meatball sandwiches, serve with pasta, or spoon onto polenta garnished with grated Parm. Starting with a leaner grind of beef helps keep too much fat from rendering into the sauce.

1 large egg

1 pound 90% lean ground beef

½ cup dried breadcrumbs

2 teaspoons Italian seasoning

1 teaspoon kosher salt

1 tablespoon olive oil

2½ cups marinara sauce (20 ounces)

1. Crack the egg into a medium bowl. Beat with a fork. Add the beef, breadcrumbs, Italian seasoning, and salt. Mix with the fork or your hands to combine. Roll the mixture into 12 meatballs.

2. Set the Instant Pot or other multicooker to Sauté and add the olive oil. When the oil is hot, add the meatballs in a single layer (you might have to perch one or two on top). Brown the meatballs for 4 minutes; there's no need to flip them. Press Cancel.

3. Add the marinara sauce. Lock the lid and set to cook on high pressure for 5 minutes.

4. When cooking is complete, press Cancel and let the pressure release naturally for 10 minutes. Carefully quick-release the remaining pressure and remove the lid. (The valve may have already floated down.) Stir gently to to unstick any meatballs and coat them in the sauce.

ROUND IT OUT Pasta, polenta, or couscous; Any Green Leaf Salad (page 193) and/or Everyday Broccoli (page 197)

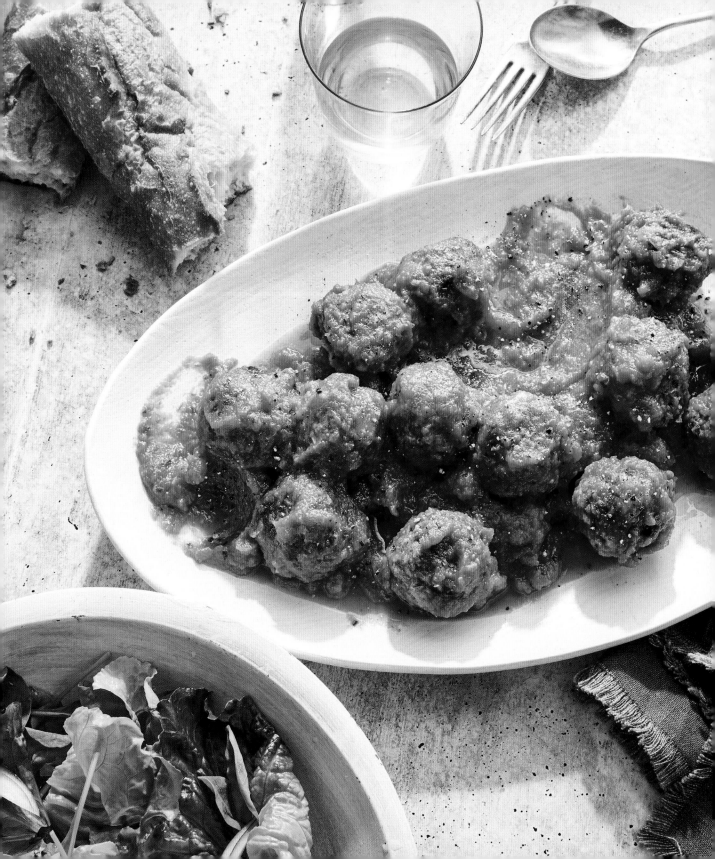

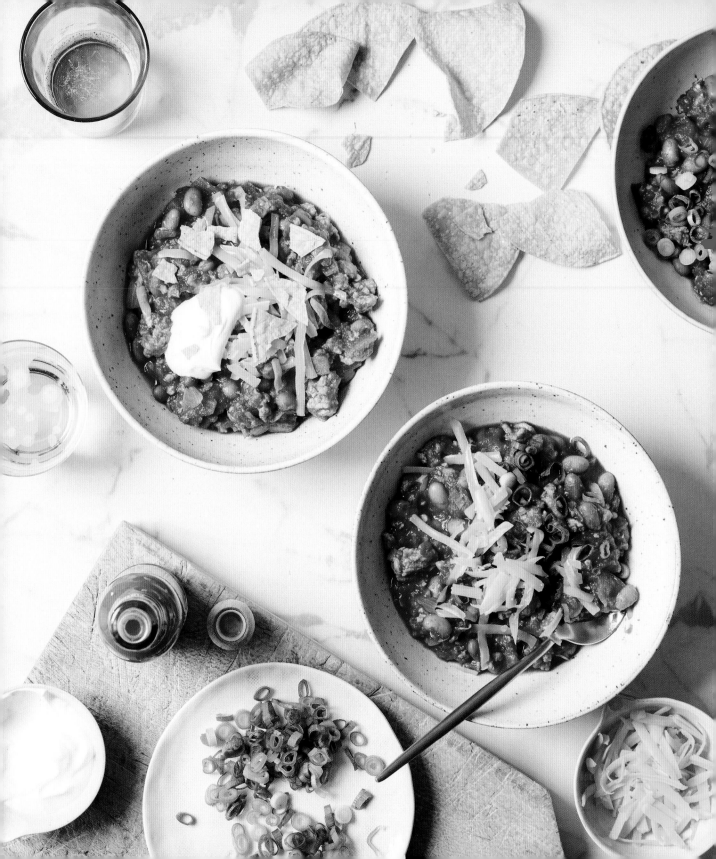

Instant Pot Turkey Chili

MAKES 4 SERVINGS

This is my favorite chili reworked for the Instant Pot, along with a few other tweaks. The recipe easily doubles (it will still fit in the Instant Pot), so consider making a big batch and freezing the leftovers. If you prefer a milder chili, dial the chili powder back to 1 teaspoon.

1 tablespoon olive oil

1 pound 93% lean ground turkey

1 yellow onion, chopped

1½ teaspoons kosher salt, divided

2 cloves garlic, roughly chopped

2 teaspoons chili powder

1 teaspoon ground cumin

½ teaspoon ground coriander

2 tablespoons tomato paste

1 28-ounce can diced tomatoes, with their juice

1 14-ounce can pinto beans, rinsed and drained

1 tablespoon maple syrup

DRESS IT UP Hot sauce, sour cream, chopped scallions, grated cheddar cheese, crushed tortilla chips

1. Set the Instant Pot or other multicooker to Sauté and add the olive oil. When the oil is hot, add the ground turkey, onion, and 1 teaspoon of the salt. Cook the turkey, breaking up the meat with a wooden spoon, until no longer pink, about 5 minutes. Stir in the garlic, chili powder, cumin, and coriander and cook for 1 minute. Add the tomato paste and cook, stirring, until it is incorporated and fragrant, about 1 minute more. Press Cancel.

2. Stir in the tomatoes, pinto beans, maple syrup, and remaining ½ teaspoon salt. Lock the lid and set to cook on high pressure for 10 minutes.

3. When cooking is complete, press Cancel and let the pressure release naturally for 10 minutes. Carefully quick-release the remaining pressure and remove the lid. Dress up the chili with any garnishes you'd like.

Instant Pot Butternut Squash and Cauliflower Curry

Frozen cauliflower and pre-cut squash make this speedy Southeast Asian–style coconut curry even more convenient. And while you can certainly eat it in a bowl as is, you'll be glad to have a bed of rice to soak up the delicious broth. Make the rice on the stove-top while the curry cooks, or heat up one of those convenient bags in the microwave.

1 tablespoon coconut oil

1½ tablespoons red curry paste

1 tablespoon finely chopped fresh ginger

1 13.5-ounce can coconut milk (well shaken)

1 pound butternut squash chunks (about 2 cups)

1 10–12-ounce bag frozen cauliflower florets

1 red bell pepper, seeded and sliced

¾ teaspoon kosher salt

2 teaspoons fish sauce, soy sauce, or tamari

Juice of ½ lime

DRESS IT UP Chopped cilantro, sriracha

1. Set the Instant Pot or other multicooker to Sauté and add the oil. When the oil is hot, add the curry paste, taking care as it will spatter a little. Stir with a wooden spoon to combine and cook until the paste darkens a touch, about 1 minute. Add the ginger and cook for 1 minute more.

2. Whisk in the coconut milk. Add the butternut squash, cauliflower florets, bell pepper, and salt and stir to combine. Lock the lid and set to cook on high pressure for 4 minutes.

3. When cooking is complete, press Cancel and carefully quick-release the pressure. Stir in the fish sauce and lime juice. Serve topped with cilantro and sriracha, if desired.

ROUND IT OUT Steamed rice

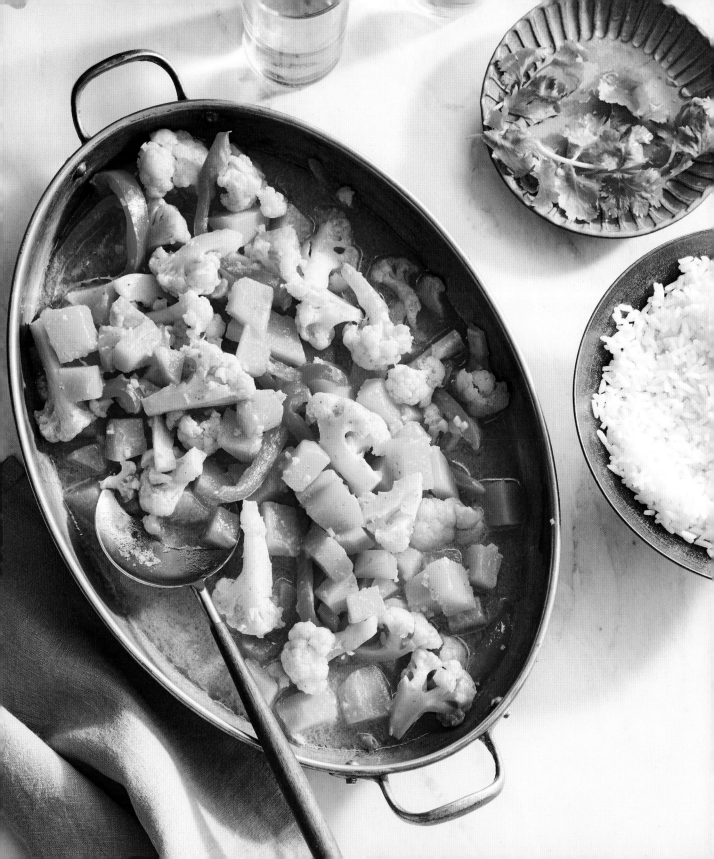

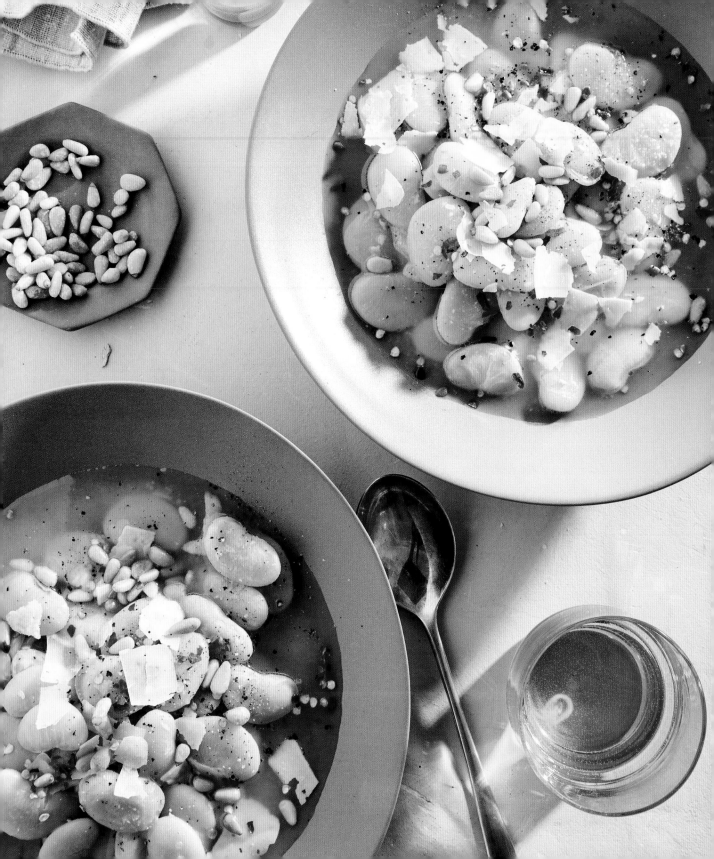

Instant Pot Creamy Butter Beans

MAKES 4 SERVINGS

Not everyone is the type of person who is happy eating a bowl of beans for dinner. But I sure am, especially when they're these lush, comforting beans finished with a flurry of tasty toppings. "Butter beans" are large lima beans; I like Bob's Red Mill brand. If you can't find butter beans, you can swap in cannellini, but add on 5 minutes of cooking time. These beans also make a terrific side dish. Just a note on all that garlic: It mellows out during the cook time, subtly flavoring the broth. There's no sharpness here.

2 tablespoons olive oil, plus more for finishing

8 cloves garlic, halved lengthwise

2 cups dried butter beans, rinsed

1½ teaspoons kosher salt

DRESS IT UP Pesto, flaky sea salt, freshly ground black pepper, toasted pine nuts, grated Parmesan cheese

1. Set the Instant Pot or other multicooker to Sauté and add the olive oil. When the oil is hot, add the garlic and cook, stirring, for 1 minute. Add the beans, taking care as it will spatter a bit. Pour in 3½ cups water and stir in the salt. Lock the lid and set to cook on high pressure for 30 minutes.

2. When cooking is complete, press Cancel and let the pressure release naturally for 10 minutes. Carefully quick-release the remaining pressure and remove the lid. Serve with a drizzle of olive oil and any of your favorite toppings.

ROUND IT OUT Any Green Leaf Salad (page 193)

Instant Pot Saucy Chicken

MAKES 4 SERVINGS

This is less of a recipe and more of a template, because making chicken with a jarred sauce in the Instant Pot is so easy and so adaptable. In any guise, this meal is a workhorse. You need chicken, a sauce, and a starch to soak up the sauce.

1½ cups sauce (see options on facing page)

1–1¼ pounds boneless, skinless chicken thighs

1 tablespoon unsalted butter (optional)

1. Pour the sauce into the Instant Pot or other multicooker. Add the chicken thighs and turn with a fork or tongs to coat. Lock the lid and set to cook on high pressure for 10 minutes.

2. When cooking is complete, press Cancel and let the pressure release naturally for 10 minutes. Carefully quick-release the remaining pressure and remove the lid. (The valve may have already floated down.) Transfer the chicken to a shallow dish.

3. If the sauce seems thin, set the Instant Pot to Sauté and let the sauce simmer for 5 to 10 minutes to thicken slightly. Press Cancel and stir in the butter, if using.

4. While the sauce is simmering, shred the chicken with 2 forks. When the sauce is ready, return the chicken to the pot and stir to combine. Serve with your choice of starch and toppers (see options on the facing page).

Sauce: Indian simmer sauce (such as Maya Kaimal brand)
Starch: Rice or naan
Topper: Sliced scallions and/or chopped cilantro

Sauce: Marinara sauce
Starch: Pasta, couscous, or crusty bread
Topper: Grated Parmesan cheese

Sauce: Tomatillo salsa (skip the optional butter)
Starch: Rice, tortillas, or tortilla chips
Topper: Slivered radishes and/or sliced scallions

Sauce: Enchilada sauce (skip the optional butter)
Starch: Rice, tortillas, or tortilla chips
Topper: Shredded cheddar cheese, cotija, and/or chopped red or white onion

Sauce: 1 cup mango chutney and ½ cup chicken broth
Starch: Rice or naan
Topper: Chopped cilantro and/or mint

Sauce: Barbecue sauce (skip the optional butter)
Starch: Sandwich rolls or buns
Topper: Shredded cabbage or Eat-with-Everything Slaw (page 196)

Slow-Cooker Big-Batch Lasagna

MAKES 8 SERVINGS

This recipe makes a large lasagna, which is great news if you're feeding a crowd and even better news if you aren't, because it freezes like a champ. Cut it into individual servings, then freeze in airtight containers and allow your future self to take a night off.

6 cups marinara sauce (48 ounces)

1 pound dry lasagna noodles

3 cups full-fat ricotta cheese (24 ounces)

2 cups shredded low-moisture mozzarella cheese (about 8 ounces)

½ cup grated Parmesan cheese (about 2 ounces), plus more for serving (optional)

MAKE IT MEATY Layer in 8 ounces browned and crumbled Italian sausage, ground beef, or ground turkey.

Slow Cooker Cooking Tip

Most slow cooker recipes give a range of cooking times since different appliances cook at slightly different rates. I typically set my slow cooker at the low end of the cooking time, check the food when the time is up, and add on more cooking time if necessary. But if you know that your slow cooker tends to be on the slower side, feel free to start on the higher end of the cook-time range. As for cooking on the High or Low setting, I decide based on when I want the meal to be completed. If I'm setting it in the morning, I typically cook it all day on Low. If it's a weekend afternoon and I'm making that evening's dinner, I'll set it on High.

1. Spread 1½ cups of the marinara sauce in the bottom of a 5- to 6-quart slow cooker. Place 3 or 4 lasagna noodles (depending on the size of the insert) on top of the sauce, breaking them as necessary to create a single layer (it's okay if the noodles overlap slightly). Dollop and spread 1 cup of the ricotta cheese over the noodles, then sprinkle with ½ cup of the mozzarella, 2 tablespoons of the Parmesan, and 1 cup sauce.

2. Arrange 3 or 4 more noodles over the sauce, followed by another 1 cup ricotta cheese, ½ cup mozzarella, 2 tablespoons Parmesan, and 1 cup sauce. Repeat with another layer of noodles, ricotta, mozzarella, Parmesan, and sauce. Then add one final layer of noodles, sauce, and mozzarella. (You might not need to use all the noodles.)

3. Cover and cook on High for 3 to 4 hours or on Low for 6 to 7 hours, until the noodles are tender.

4. Turn off the heat, remove the lid, and let the lasagna sit for 10 to 15 minutes before slicing and serving. Top with additional Parmesan, if desired.

Slow-Cooker Salmon with Lemon and Dill

MAKES 4 SERVINGS

The slow cooker is a truly foolproof way to turn out fish that is delicate, succulent, and extremely flavorful. To ensure that you can get the salmon out of the slow cooker without it completely falling apart, line your slow cooker with aluminum foil. Once the fish is cooked, lift it up by the foil, rather than trying to grab it with a spatula or tongs.

2 lemons

1 1½-pound skin-on salmon fillet

½ cup white wine

¾ teaspoon kosher salt

Freshly ground black pepper to taste

2 tablespoons chopped dill

1. Line a 5- to 6-quart slow cooker with a piece of aluminum foil that is long enough to come up the sides of the insert by a few inches. Thinly slice 1½ of the lemons and juice the remaining half. Lay half of the lemon slices in the bottom of the slow cooker, then lay the salmon on top, skin side down.

2. Add the wine, ½ cup water, and lemon juice to the slow cooker. Season the salmon with the salt and plenty of pepper. Sprinkle the salmon with the chopped dill and top with the remaining lemon slices. Cook on Low for 1½ to 2 hours, depending on how well done you like your salmon. To check doneness, use a sharp knife to peek inside the middle of the fillet.

3. Serve immediately, or cool and refrigerate to eat chilled later.

ROUND IT OUT Everyday Broccoli (page 197), Asparagus with Garlicky Mayo (page 210), or Quinoa Pilaf (page 222)

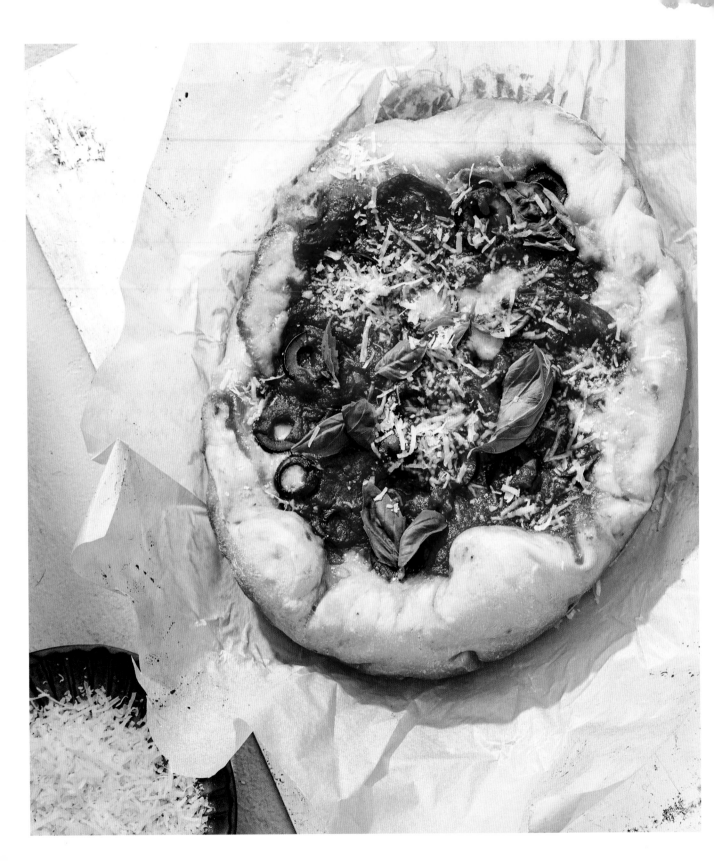

Slow-Cooker Deep-Dish Pizza

MAKES 4 SERVINGS

This recipe is a riff on Chicago-style deep-dish pizza, with the cheese hiding underneath the toppings and the sauce. Don't skip the paper towel trick—a layer of paper towels in between the insert and the lid absorbs moisture so your crust won't get soggy. If it gets saturated before the cooking time is up, just replace it with fresh paper towels. Let the pizza dough rest at room temperature for 30 minutes before starting the recipe.

1 pound white pizza dough, thawed if frozen

2 cups shredded low-moisture mozzarella cheese (about 8 ounces)

Optional toppings: 8 ounces crumbled cooked Italian sausage, sliced pepperoni, sliced olives, or sliced bell peppers

1 cup pizza or marinara sauce

DRESS IT UP Grated Parmesan cheese, basil leaves

1. On a large sheet of parchment paper, stretch the pizza dough into a circle or an oval (depending on the shape of your 5- to 6-quart slow cooker) that is about 2 inches bigger all around than the insert of your slow cooker. Use the edges of the parchment to lift and then lower the crust (still on the parchment) into the slow cooker. Gently tug and stretch the dough up the sides of the insert.

2. Scatter the cheese over the surface of the pizza dough. Add any additional toppings over the cheese, then spread the tomato sauce over the toppings. Again, lift and stretch the edges of the crust so that it reaches above the filling.

3. Cover the top of the slow cooker with a long piece of paper towel, then place the lid over the paper towel and pull it tight.

4. Cook the pizza on High for 2 to 3 hours or on Low for 4 to 5 hours, until the crust is golden brown but still tender enough to cut. When you are ready to serve, use the edges of the parchment paper to lift the pizza out of the slow cooker. Let sit for 5 to 10 minutes before cutting into quarters. Sprinkle with Parmesan cheese and basil, if desired.

Slow-Cooker Beef Ragu

MAKES 8 SERVINGS

Few dishes can compare to a comforting bowl of long-braised beef ragu. It's the kind of recipe slow cookers were made for—simmering all day long, making your house smell amazing, and resulting in a dish that is as tender and flavorful as can be. While it's hard to resist digging in right away (and it's okay if you do!), this ragu is even better the next day. Once it's cool, store it in the fridge overnight. The next day, scoop out and discard the layer of fat on the surface before reheating.

½ cup red wine

½ cup low-sodium beef broth

1 28-ounce can crushed tomatoes

1 6-ounce can tomato paste

1 yellow onion, chopped

3 cloves garlic, finely chopped

1 celery stalk, chopped

1 carrot, chopped

3 teaspoons kosher salt, divided

2 sprigs thyme or 1 teaspoon dried thyme (optional)

1 sprig sage or 1 teaspoon dried sage (optional)

1 Parmesan cheese rind (optional)

2 pounds bone-in beef short ribs

Freshly ground black pepper to taste

Cooked pasta, polenta, or rice, for serving

1. Whisk together the wine, broth, crushed tomatoes, and tomato paste in a 6-quart slow cooker. Stir in the onion, garlic, celery, carrot, and 2 teaspoons of the salt. Add the thyme, sage, and Parmesan rind, if using.

2. Season the short ribs with the remaining 1 teaspoon salt and a generous grinding of pepper and add them to the slow cooker.

3. Cover and cook on Low for 7 to 9 hours, until the meat is very tender and pulls away from the bone.

4. Transfer the short ribs to a large platter or bowl, then shred the meat and discard the bones. Discard the herb sprigs and Parmesan rind, if using, and stir the meat back into the sauce.

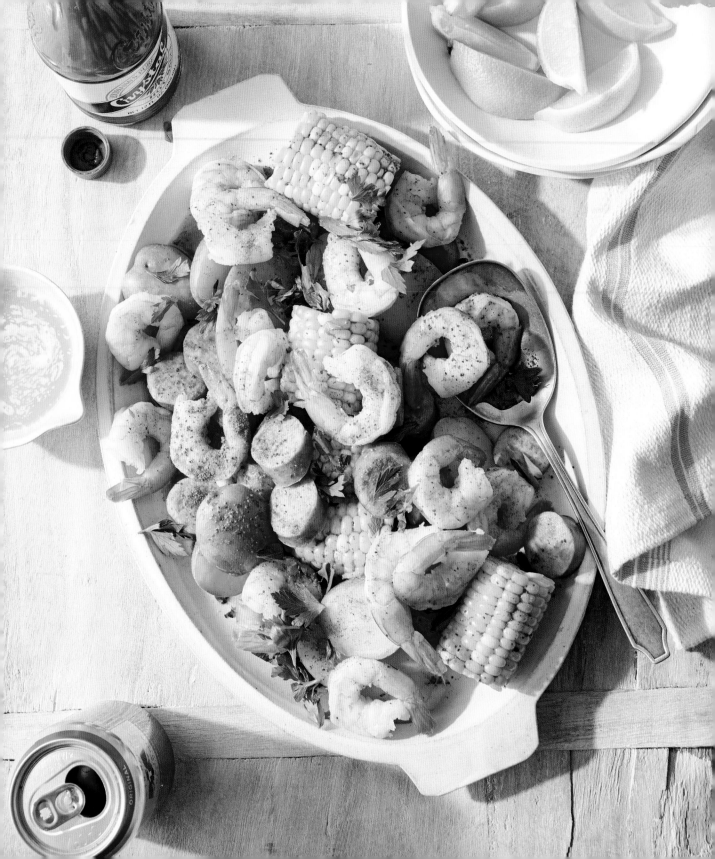

Slow-Cooker Shrimp Boil

MAKES 6 TO 8 SERVINGS

This classic shrimp boil—a combination of fresh shrimp, potatoes, corn, and sausage all cooked in a flavorful broth—is a complete one-pot meal that's perfect for feeding a crowd. Buy the largest shrimp you can find for this recipe, so they don't get lost in the mix.

1½ pounds small red potatoes, halved

1 pound smoked sausage (such as andouille or kielbasa), cut into 1-inch pieces

3 ears corn, shucked and cut crosswise into thirds

6 cloves garlic, peeled and lightly smashed

¼ cup Old Bay seasoning, plus more for serving

1 lemon, halved, plus additional wedges for serving

1½ pounds raw large shrimp (16–20 per pound), peeled and deveined, tails on

Melted butter and hot sauce, for serving

DRESS IT UP Chopped parsley, freshly ground black pepper

1. Arrange the potatoes in the bottom of a 6-quart or larger slow cooker. Add the sausage, corn, and garlic. Sprinkle the Old Bay evenly over the ingredients, squeeze the lemon halves into the slow cooker, then toss in the squeezed halves.

2. Pour 5 to 6 cups water over the ingredients, adding enough so that it comes about halfway up the corn. Do not stir.

3. Cover and cook on Low for 5 to 6 hours, until the potatoes are tender when pierced with a fork.

4. Increase the temperature to High, add the shrimp, stir gently, cover, and cook just until the shrimp are opaque, 10 to 15 minutes.

5. Using a slotted spoon, transfer the contents of the slow cooker to a large platter or individual serving bowls. Drizzle everything with some of the cooking liquid and sprinkle with more Old Bay, plus parsley and pepper, if desired. Serve with lemon wedges, melted butter, and hot sauce.

Slow-Cooker Ropa Vieja

MAKES 5 TO 6 SERVINGS

This traditionally Cuban dish gets its name from the use of flank steak, which—when shredded—has long, ropey fibers. (Ropa vieja translates to "old clothes.") Hanger steak, chuck roast, top round, brisket, or skirt steak would all produce equally delicious results.

1 28-ounce can diced tomatoes, with their juice

2 red bell peppers, seeded and thinly sliced

1 medium onion, chopped

4 cloves garlic, finely chopped

1 jalapeño pepper, thinly sliced

1 teaspoon ground cumin

½ teaspoon dried oregano

1 2-pound flank steak

2 teaspoons kosher salt

Freshly ground black pepper to taste

½ cup pitted green olives, roughly chopped

3 tablespoons capers, drained

½ cup coarsely chopped cilantro

Steamed white rice or warm tortillas, for serving

1. Combine the diced tomatoes, bell peppers, onion, garlic, jalapeño, cumin, and oregano in a 5- to 6-quart slow cooker. Season both sides of the flank steak with the salt and plenty of pepper. Lay the flank steak on top of the vegetables, cover, and cook on High for 5 to 6 hours or on Low for 7 to 8 hours, until the meat is very tender.

2. Transfer the meat to a cutting board and shred with 2 forks.

3. Stir the olives, capers, and cilantro into the sauce in the slow cooker. Return the meat to the sauce and stir to combine.

4. Use a slotted spoon to transfer the meat to bowls, and serve with steamed rice or warm tortillas.

Ingredient Tip

To quickly slice bell peppers, stand them upright and slice down around the pepper, about a half-inch from the stem on all sides. You'll miss most of the seeds this way. Slice out the ribs and flick out any stray seeds.

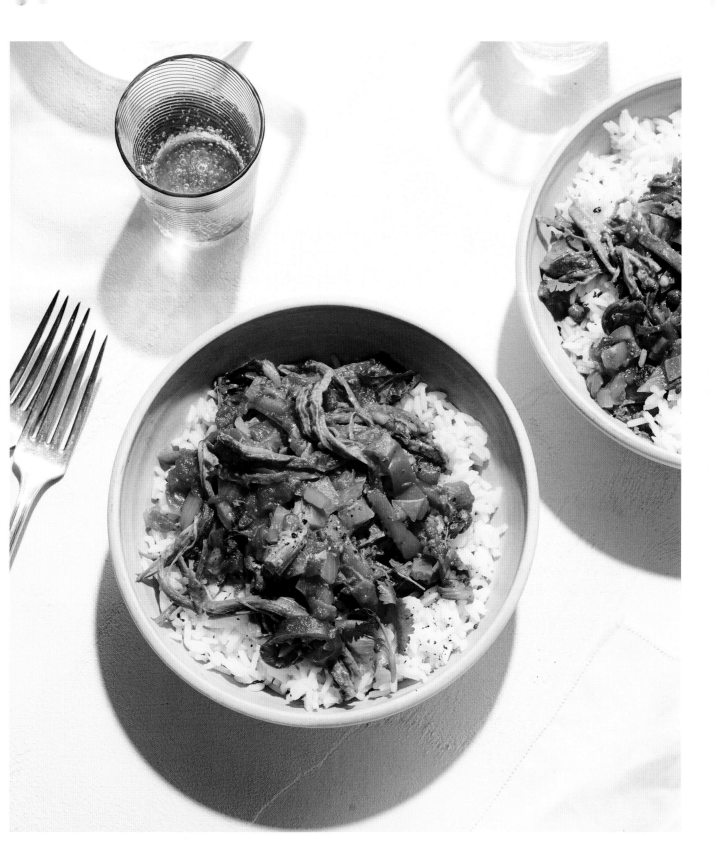

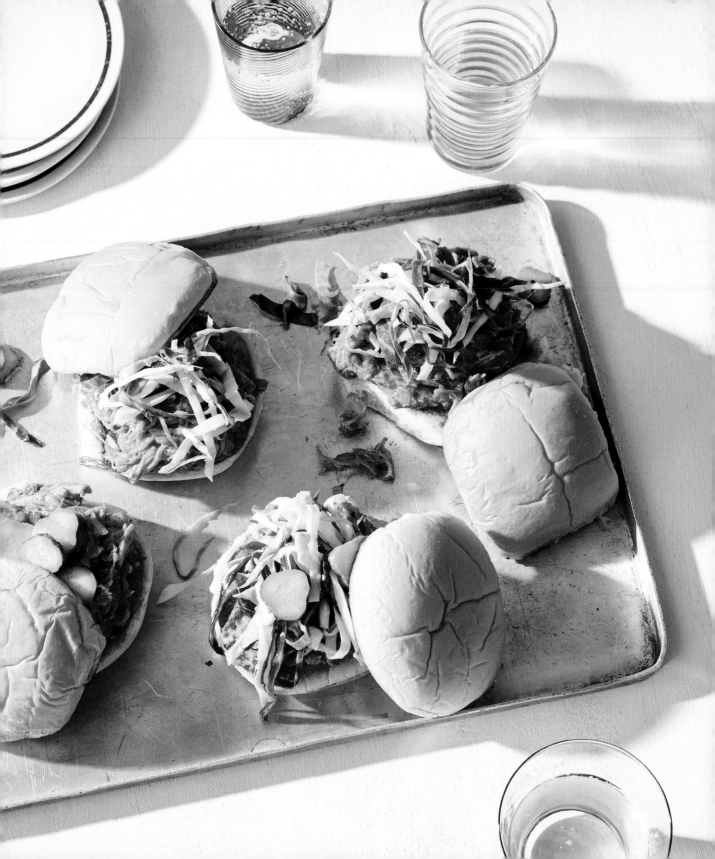

Slow-Cooker BBQ Pulled Pork Sandwiches

MAKES 8 TO 10 SERVINGS

All it takes to turn out truly amazing pulled pork is a handful of ingredients and half a day or so to let your slow cooker do what it does best: braise that meat low and slow. While serving this BBQ heaped on potato rolls with slaw and pickles is traditional, it also makes for really delicious tacos. Just tuck pickled onions, shredded pepper Jack cheese, and cilantro into warm tortillas.

1 small onion, finely chopped

¾ cup ketchup

¼ cup apple cider vinegar

3 tablespoons tomato paste

1 teaspoon sweet paprika

1 teaspoon garlic powder

1 teaspoon ground mustard

1 teaspoon ground cumin

1 3–4-pound boneless pork shoulder

1½ teaspoons kosher salt, plus more to taste

Freshly ground black pepper to taste

Potato buns, for serving

DRESS IT UP Eat-with-Everything Slaw (page 196), pickles

1. Combine the onion, ketchup, apple cider vinegar, tomato paste, and spices in a 5- to 6-quart slow cooker. Season the pork shoulder with the salt and plenty of pepper. Lay the seasoned pork shoulder in the slow cooker, cover, and cook on High for 5 to 6 hours or on Low for 8 to 10 hours, until the meat is very tender.

2. Transfer the meat to a cutting board or bowl and shred with 2 forks. Return the meat to the sauce. Season with additional salt and pepper to taste. Serve on potato buns with slaw and/or pickles, if desired.

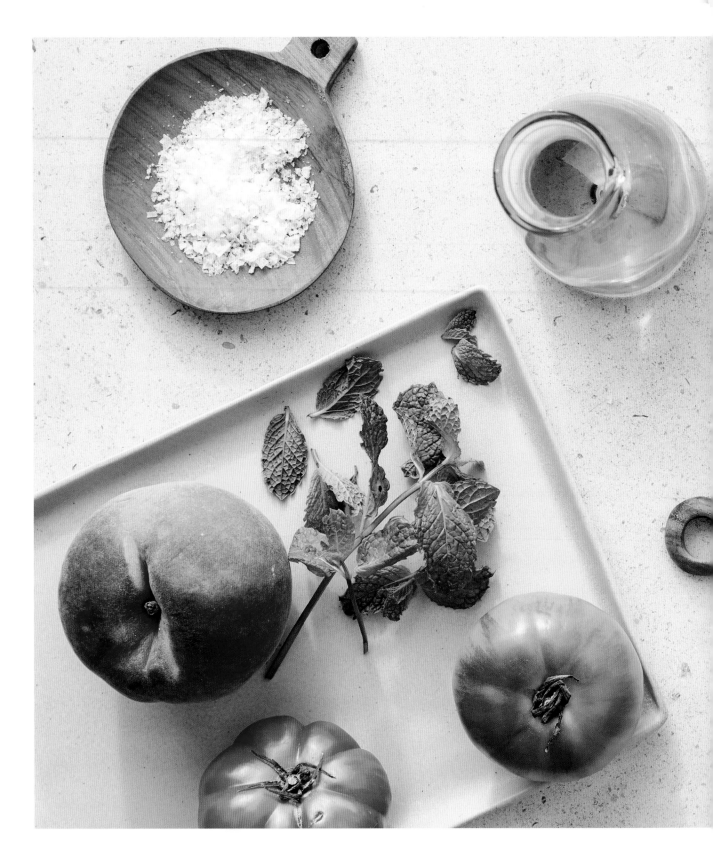

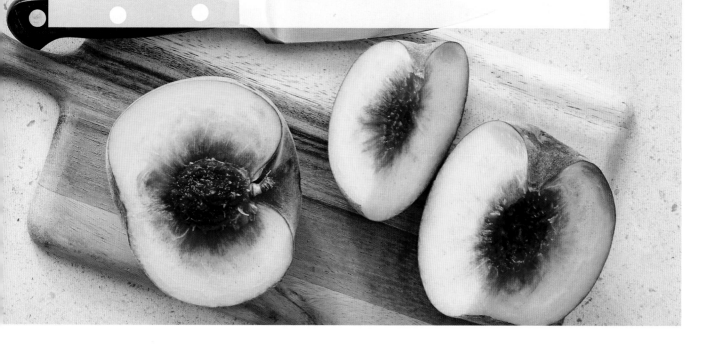

BARE MINIMUM
Sides

Easy Add-Ons to Round Out Dinner

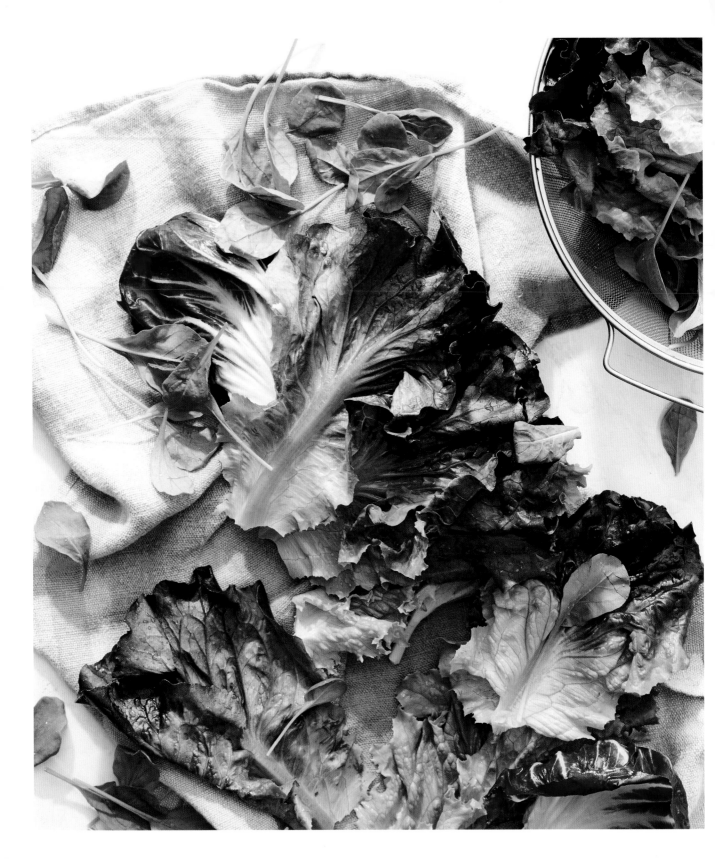

Any Green Leaf Salad

MAKES 4 SERVINGS

I am a firm believer that a leafy green salad rounds out most meals. And, happily, this salad takes 5 minutes (or less!) to put together if you have washed greens on hand. (See page 195 for washing basics.)

I like salad dressings as much as the next gal, and they certainly aren't hard to make and will last in the refrigerator for several days. However, I am not quite as dedicated to making salad dressings in advance as I am to washing greens ahead of time. And for an everyday salad, I find this mix-it-all-in-a-bowl method ideal.

Some people advocate for dressing salads with acid before olive oil, but I prefer the oil-first method. I think of salad greens as any other veggie—so just as I would for, say, steamed cauliflower or potatoes, I drizzle with olive oil, season with salt, and spritz with lemon. But, have fun! Experiment! There is no right or wrong here.

In my house, we don't like our salads very acidic. With some meals I do want a bracing salad with lots of sour bite. But usually I prefer a gentler salad, probably influenced by my teenager who favors mild leafy greens. I call for a range of acid here; feel free to add even more if you'd like.

If you make salads frequently, you may not need to measure the ingredients and can just eyeball them instead. When in doubt, taste, adjust, and taste again.

5 cups salad greens, torn into bite-sized pieces if large, including any or all: romaine lettuce, red leaf lettuce, green leaf lettuce, arugula, spinach, spring mix, baby kale, mesclun mix

1½ tablespoons olive oil

¼ teaspoon kosher salt, or more to taste

Freshly ground black pepper to taste (optional)

1–2 teaspoons lemon juice or vinegar (rice, apple cider, red wine, white wine, or balsamic)

Pile the salad greens in a large bowl. Drizzle on the olive oil and sprinkle on the salt. Add the pepper, if using. Toss gently with your clean hands or tongs. Add the lemon juice or vinegar and toss again. Taste. Add more oil, acid, salt, or pepper, if desired.

BASIC KALE SALAD

What about a kale salad, you ask, made with curly kale or lacinato kale? Those are green leaves too, after all! The basic principle is the same, but since kale is less tender than lettuce it needs a little more attention. To prepare kale, remove and discard the thick stems. Tear the leaves into bite-sized pieces to make 5 cups. Drizzle with 2 tablespoons olive oil and sprinkle on ½ teaspoon kosher salt. Using your clean hands, rub the oil and salt into the leaves until all the leaves are coated. This helps tenderize the leaves. Add 2 teaspoons lemon juice and pepper to taste, if desired. Toss again, with your hands or tongs, and taste. Add up to ¼ teaspoon more salt if you'd like. This salad can sit for up to a half hour at room temperature before serving.

HOW TO WASH AND STORE LEAFY GREENS

If you have to wash lettuce leaves every time you want a salad, it's all too easy to just skip the whole thing. One option is to buy prewashed greens in a plastic clamshell or bag. I do that occasionally, but much less frequently than I used to, as I'm trying to reduce the amount of plastic I bring into my kitchen. Instead, I wash a head of lettuce or a bunch of kale soon after I bring it home from the grocery store or farmers' market and store it for simple salads over the next several days. Here's how:

Soak the leaves in water in a big salad spinner (a kitchen essential if you want to eat more salads!) for a minute or two, swishing with your hands to dislodge any dirt. Be sure not to fill the spinner more than three-quarters full; if you have more greens than that, you'll need to wash them in multiple batches. You may need to rinse the leaves more than once before spinning them dry; if you see sand or dirt in the water when you drain it, rinse the lettuce or kale again. (I find that if I buy greens from the grocery store, I usually need to wash them only once. If I bring greens home from the farmers' market, it takes two or three times.) Once the greens are clean, place a paper towel over them, and spin away. I find it challenging to get the leaves completely dry in the salad spinner, so after several spins I transfer them to a dish towel(s) in a single layer to air-dry for 10 to 15 minutes. To store, place a paper towel in a zip-top plastic bag or large storage container. Add the almost-completely-dry greens. It's okay if they're still *slightly* damp since the paper towel will absorb extra moisture. If using a bag, gently push down to release any air, seal, and refrigerate. The lettuce or kale will keep for nearly a week in the fridge. You can wash and store tender herbs like parsley, cilantro, basil, and mint the same way.

SALAD ADD-INS

It's easy to jazz up your green salad with a handful of one or more of these options:

- Grated carrot
- Cucumber half-moons
- Radish half-moons
- Halved cherry tomatoes
- Shredded cabbage
- Thinly sliced scallions
- Thinly sliced red onion
- Leaves of tender herbs
- Grated Parmesan, pecorino Romano, or Manchego cheese; crumbled feta or blue cheese (especially nice on kale salads)
- Raisins
- Dried cranberries or cherries
- Toasted chopped nuts or seeds (including walnuts, hazelnuts, pecans, pistachios, almonds, pepitas, and sunflower seeds)

Eat-with-Everything Slaw

This hearty salad is incredibly versatile. It adds crunch to tacos (and you see a variation of it on a couple of the taco recipes in this book), snap to sandwiches, and veggie power to just about any other meal. My go-to acid here is rice vinegar, since it's a bit less sharp than other vinegars or citrus, but use whatever you prefer or have on hand. The recipe works with any type of cabbage: green, purple, savoy, or napa.

4 cups shredded cabbage (about 12 ounces)

2 tablespoons rice vinegar

¾ teaspoon kosher salt, plus more to taste

Pinch granulated sugar

Combine all the ingredients in a medium bowl. Toss to coat the cabbage. Let sit for 10 to 30 minutes, tossing occasionally. Taste before serving and add a little more salt, if desired.

Cooking Tip

You can store leftover slaw (except for one made with more tender napa cabbage) for up to 24 hours in the fridge. Sprinkle with a little additional salt before serving.

Everyday Broccoli

MAKES 4 SERVINGS

Whoever compared eating broccoli to a distasteful activity clearly hadn't eaten properly cooked broccoli, possibly the greatest-of-all-time veggie. Roasted broccoli is delish, but I find myself gravitating to this simple yet lush boiled broccoli dressed with garlicky olive oil. I prefer broccoli boiled Italian-style, in well-salted water and cooked past tender-crisp to plain old tender (but never mushy!). I often cook the broccoli first when I'm making dinner and serve it at room temperature when the rest of the meal is ready. This is an especially smart strategy when making pasta since you can scoop the cooked broccoli out of the boiling water and add the pasta right after.

Kosher salt, for the cooking water and seasoning

1 bunch broccoli, cut into slender florets with 1–2-inch stems

3 tablespoons olive oil

2 cloves garlic, thinly sliced

⅛ teaspoon crushed red pepper (optional)

DRESS IT UP Flaky sea salt

Cooking Tip

To make this even easier, skip the garlic oil and just drizzle the cooked broccoli with olive oil and sprinkle with sea salt.

1. Bring a large pot of well-salted water to a boil. Add the broccoli and cook until it's tender to your liking, 4 to 5 minutes. Drain in a colander or fish the broccoli out with a spider or slotted spoon and transfer to a shallow serving dish.

2. Heat the olive oil in a small skillet over medium-low heat. Add the sliced garlic, a large pinch of salt, and the crushed red pepper, if using. Cook until the garlic is tender and no more than lightly browned, 4 to 5 minutes. Pour the garlic oil over the broccoli in the serving dish. Top with flaky sea salt, if desired.

Spicy Oven Fries

MAKES 4 SERVINGS

Alas, the very best oven fries—the crispiest, the most golden—require first blanching and drying the potatoes before roasting them. That's more work than I want to do on a weeknight. But these full-flavored numbers are a close second. In this variation on a recipe my mom used to make (too infrequently as far as I was concerned), I've upped the spices and swapped in nutritional yeast for her grated Parm. The nutritional yeast is full of B vitamins and iron, and I'm always looking for ways to make good use of my stash.

2 tablespoons nutritional yeast

1 teaspoon kosher salt

1 teaspoon dried oregano

1 teaspoon chili powder

2 pounds potatoes (red, russet, or Yukon Gold), cut into wedges

2 tablespoons olive oil

Ketchup, for dipping (optional)

1. Preheat the oven to 425°F. Line a rimmed baking sheet with parchment paper.

2. In a large bowl, stir together the nutritional yeast, salt, oregano, and chili powder. Add the potatoes and drizzle in the olive oil. Toss to coat. Transfer the potatoes to the prepared baking sheet and spread into a single layer.

3. Bake for 30 minutes, flip, and bake for another 10 to 15 minutes, until golden. Serve with ketchup, if desired.

Ingredient Tip

If you don't have nutritional yeast, use grated Parmesan or pecorino cheese.

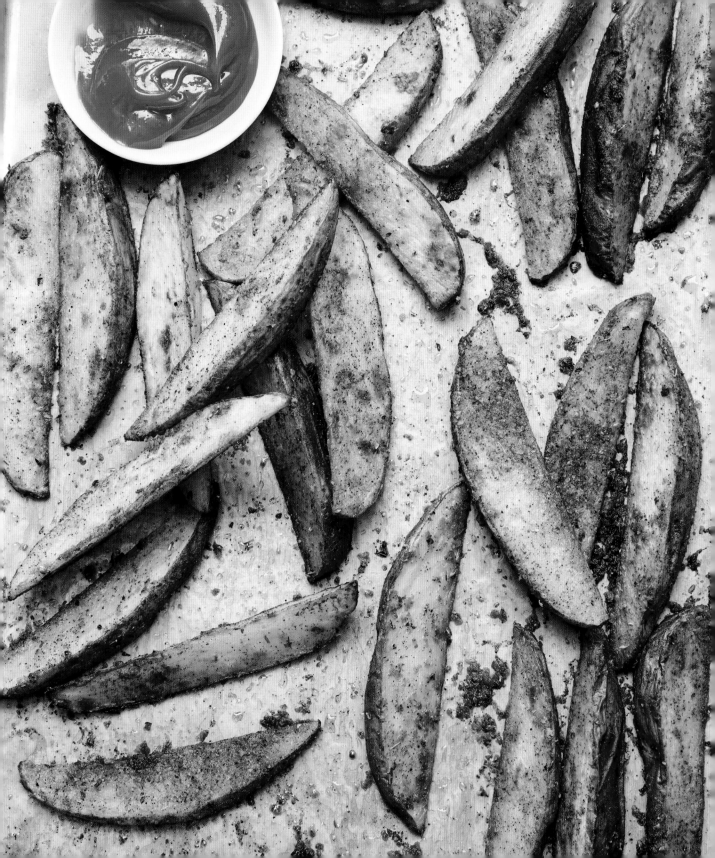

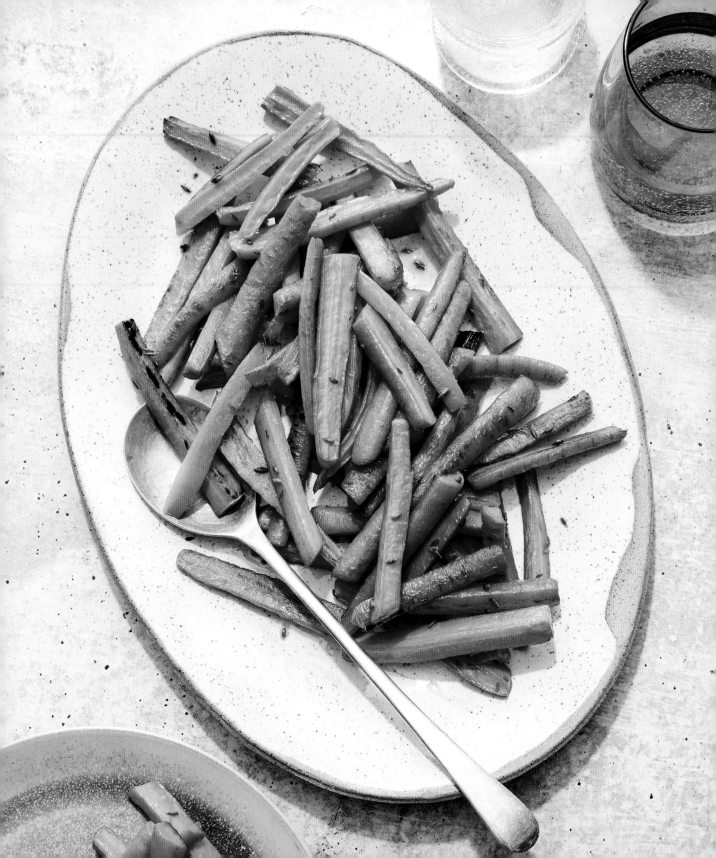

Peels-On Cumin-Roasted Carrots

MAKES 4 SERVINGS

The trick to perfectly roasted carrots—tender, yet caramelized—is to cover the baking sheet with aluminum foil for the first 15 minutes of baking time. This will partially steam the carrots so they're yielding, not woody. To me, cumin seeds make these carrots irresistible, but you can skip them if you prefer.

1 pound carrots, scrubbed and trimmed

1 tablespoon olive oil

1 teaspoon kosher salt

1 teaspoon cumin seeds

DRESS IT UP Chopped parsley or cilantro

1. Preheat the oven to 425°F. Line a rimmed baking sheet with parchment paper.

2. Cut the carrots into sticks that are about even in length and width. Place on the prepared baking sheet. Toss with the olive oil, salt, and cumin seeds. Cover the pan tightly with aluminum foil and bake for 15 minutes. Carefully remove the foil (it will be steamy in there!) and continue roasting until the carrots are tender and browned, even burnt in some spots, another 25 to 30 minutes. Top with chopped parsley or cilantro, if desired.

White Beans with Sage

MAKES 2 TO 3 SERVINGS

Serve this as a side with any grilled meat. Or, pile it on top of thick slices of toast for a light supper in its own right. This recipe doubles easily.

2 tablespoons olive oil, plus more for drizzling

1 lightly packed tablespoon chopped fresh sage

1 15-ounce can cannellini beans, rinsed and drained

2 tablespoons white wine, or 1 tablespoon lemon juice plus 1 tablespoon water

½ teaspoon kosher salt

Flaky sea salt to taste

1. Heat the olive oil in a medium skillet over medium heat. Add the sage and cook until fragrant, about 1 minute.

2. Add the beans, taking care since they will likely spatter when hitting the oil. Stir to coat. Add the wine and salt. Using the back of a wooden spoon, mash about half the beans and stir until the beans have a creamy texture, about 2 minutes. If the dish seems dry at any point, stir in a tablespoon or two of water. Serve the beans topped with a generous drizzle of olive oil and a sprinkle of flaky sea salt.

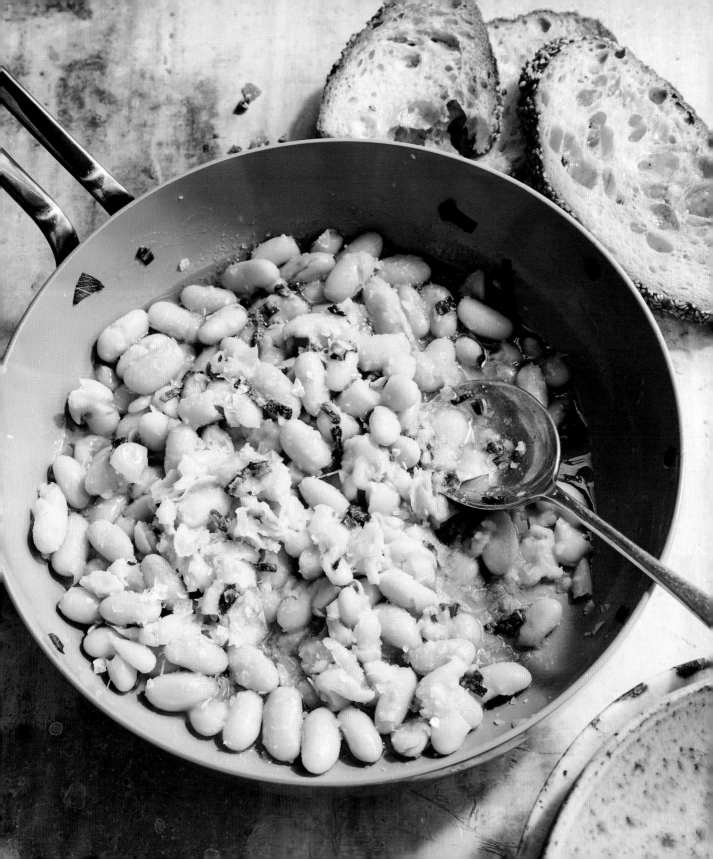

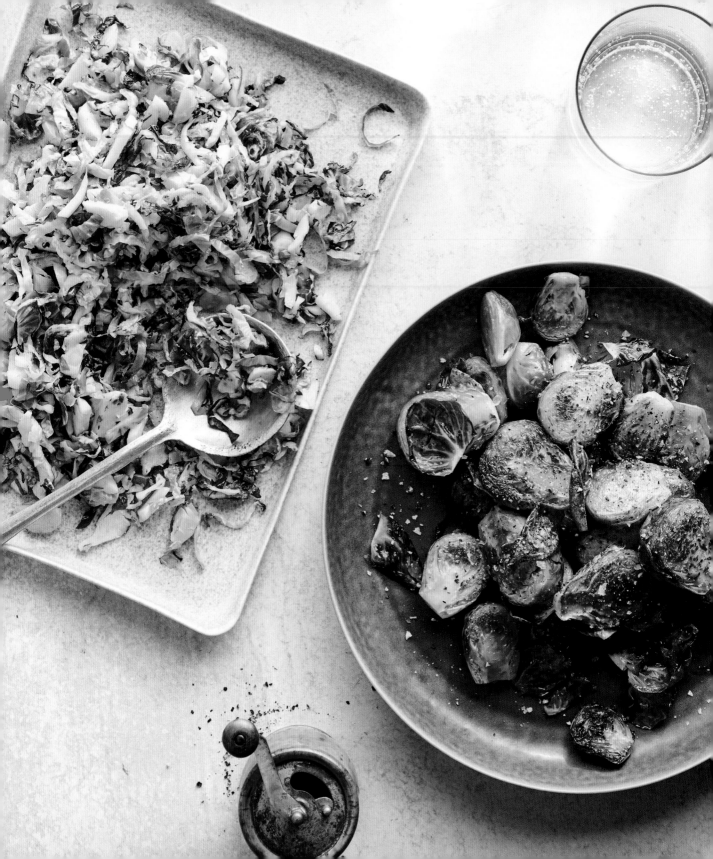

Two Ways with Roasted Brussels Sprouts

Harness the magical powers of high-heat roasting to bring out this veggie's nutty sweetness.

ROASTED SHREDDED BRUSSELS SPROUTS

MAKES 4 SERVINGS

Start with a bag or container of sliced sprouts. Or, to slice whole brussels sprouts, trim the bottom and cut a thin slice from one of the sides. Place the sprout on the flat side, and cut into thin slices.

12 ounces thinly sliced brussels sprouts (about 5 cups)

2 tablespoons olive oil

½ teaspoon kosher salt, plus more if desired

2 teaspoons sherry vinegar

1. Preheat the oven to 425°F. Line a rimmed baking sheet with parchment paper.

2. Put the sliced brussels sprouts on the prepared baking sheet and toss with the olive oil and salt. Spread in an even layer. (It's okay if some of the sprouts are on top of each other.) Roast until browned in spots, 15 to 17 minutes, stirring after 10 minutes. Stir in the vinegar. Taste for seasoning and add more salt, if desired.

SPICY-SWEET ROASTED BRUSSELS SPROUTS

MAKES 4 SERVINGS

You can make hot honey by simmering honey and hot sauce, but I like the widely available brand Mike's Hot Honey. It adds pizzazz to pizza, biscuits, and veggies—especially roasted carrots and, here, brussels sprouts. If you aren't a fan of spice, just use regular honey.

2 tablespoons olive oil

1 tablespoon hot honey

1 pound brussels sprouts, trimmed and halved (or quartered if large)

½ teaspoon kosher salt

Flaky sea salt and freshly ground black pepper to taste

1. Preheat the oven to 425°F. Line a rimmed baking sheet with parchment paper.

2. Mix the olive oil and honey in a large bowl. Add the brussels sprouts and salt and toss to coat.

3. Spread out the sprouts in a single layer on the prepared baking sheet, scraping any leftover oil and honey out of the bowl with a silicone spatula onto the sprouts. Bake until tender and browned, about 25 minutes. Season with flaky sea salt and pepper.

Two Ways with Cauliflower Rice

CHEESY CAULIFLOWER RICE

MAKES 3 TO 4 SERVINGS

Some people eat cauliflower rice to reduce their carb intake. I like it because it's a speedy way to get a veggie on the table (see Dinner Rule #1, page 23). And I don't mind wielding plenty of butter and cheese to boost the flavor. The strategy has been successful: My cauliflower-averse teenager ate almost half of this recipe the first time I made it.

2 tablespoons unsalted butter, divided

1 12-ounce bag frozen cauliflower rice

¾ teaspoon kosher salt

¼ cup grated Parmesan cheese (about 1 ounce), plus more for serving

Freshly ground black pepper to taste

Heat 1 tablespoon of the butter in a medium nonstick skillet over medium heat. Add the cauliflower rice, cover, and cook for 5 minutes. Stir in the salt, cover again, and cook for another 5 minutes. Stir in the remaining 1 tablespoon butter, the Parmesan cheese, and plenty of pepper. Serve topped with more cheese and pepper.

SESAME-SOY CAULIFLOWER RICE

MAKES 3 TO 4 SERVINGS

To put it kindly, I would describe cauliflower rice as neutral in flavor. In this recipe, it positively soaks up soy sauce, making for a deliciously salty, can't-stop-eating side.

1 tablespoon toasted sesame oil

1 12-ounce bag frozen cauliflower rice

2 tablespoons soy sauce or tamari, divided

1 scallion, trimmed and chopped (optional)

Heat the sesame oil in a medium nonstick skillet over medium heat. Add the cauliflower rice and 1 tablespoon of the soy sauce. Cover and cook, stirring once or twice, for 8 minutes. Stir in the remaining 1 tablespoon soy sauce. Continue to cook, uncovered, stirring occasionally, until the soy sauce has soaked in and the cauliflower rice is golden and crisp in places. Stir in the scallion, if using, and serve.

All-Purpose Yogurt Dip

MAKES BIG DOLLOPS FOR 4 PEOPLE

Okay, this recipe can't wash the dishes for you, but it can do just about anything else. Use it as a dip for veggies or chips, smear it on a serving dish as a bed for roasted vegetables, or dollop it on sautéed ground meat or grilled chicken breasts.

1 5-ounce container plain whole-milk Greek yogurt (about ⅔ cup)

1 tablespoon olive oil

¼ teaspoon kosher salt

⅛ teaspoon onion powder

⅛ teaspoon garlic powder

Freshly ground black pepper to taste

Mix all of the ingredients in a small bowl. Refrigerate, covered, for up to 24 hours.

Asparagus with Garlicky Mayo

MAKES 4 SERVINGS

I love simply cooked asparagus, which I then drag through copious amounts of a bright, creamy sauce. The key here is to cook the asparagus just until it's tender, so you get that lovely snap when you bite into it.

3 tablespoons mayonnaise

1 clove garlic

½ teaspoon lemon juice

Kosher salt

1 bunch asparagus, woody ends snapped off

1. Put the mayonnaise in a small bowl. Using a Microplane grater, carefully grate the garlic into the mayo. (If you don't have a Microplane, buy one! But, in the meantime, you can use a garlic press, or chop the garlic very, very finely until it's almost a paste.) Stir in the lemon juice and a pinch of salt. Cover and refrigerate until ready to serve, up to 2 hours.

2. Bring about 2 inches water to a boil in a large skillet. Season generously with salt. Add the asparagus and cook until just tender, 2 to 4 minutes, depending on the size of the spears. Using tongs, transfer to a plate. Serve with the garlicky mayo.

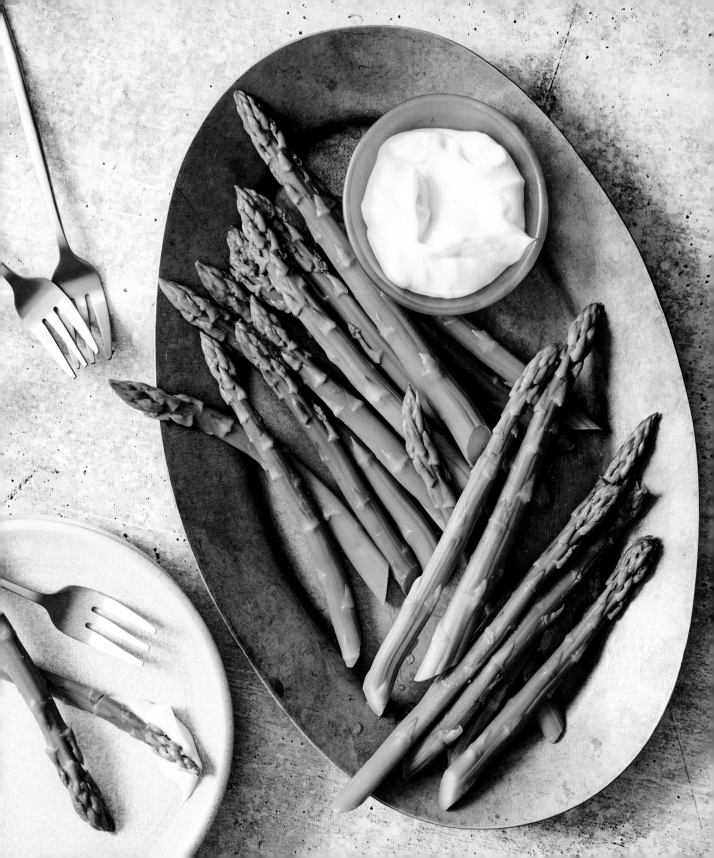

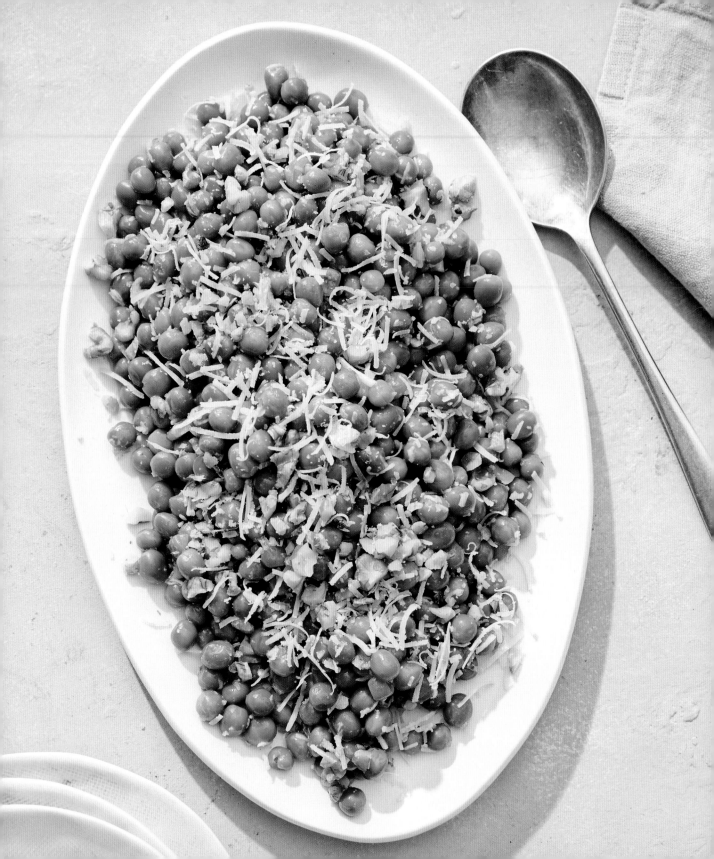

Peas with Walnuts and Parm

MAKES 4 SERVINGS

Confession: Peas are probably my least favorite veggie. But I more than tolerate them in this crunchy, cheesy dish (and my husband inhales them).

1 10-ounce bag frozen peas

2 tablespoons olive oil

¼ cup finely chopped walnuts

¼ cup grated Parmesan cheese (about 1 ounce)

¼ teaspoon kosher salt

1. Cook the peas on the stove-top according to the package directions, making sure not to overcook them. They should be bright green and just tender. Drain and return to the pot.

2. Add the olive oil and stir gently to combine. Stir in the walnuts, cheese, and salt.

Fennel-Roasted Cabbage

MAKES 4 SERVINGS

Roasting shredded cabbage is such a great way to use up the last of a head! (They often seem never-ending . . .) I sometimes like to roast cabbage until it's really browned and crispy, but this version has a bit more give: some crunchy bits, but also softer, more succulent pockets. If you want more crispiness, just keep it in the oven longer. I love the slight licorice flavor the fennel seeds give the cabbage—it's such a big flavor boost for so little effort. But, of course, if you don't like or have fennel seeds, simply leave them out.

6 cups shredded cabbage (about 1 pound)

2 tablespoons olive oil

1 teaspoon kosher salt

1 teaspoon fennel seeds

1. Preheat the oven to 425°F. Line a rimmed baking sheet with parchment paper.

2. Toss the cabbage, olive oil, salt, and fennel seeds together on the prepared baking sheet. Spread into an even layer and roast until the cabbage is crispy to your liking, 20 to 30 minutes depending on your preference and how thick the cabbage was sliced to begin with. Stir once halfway through the cooking time.

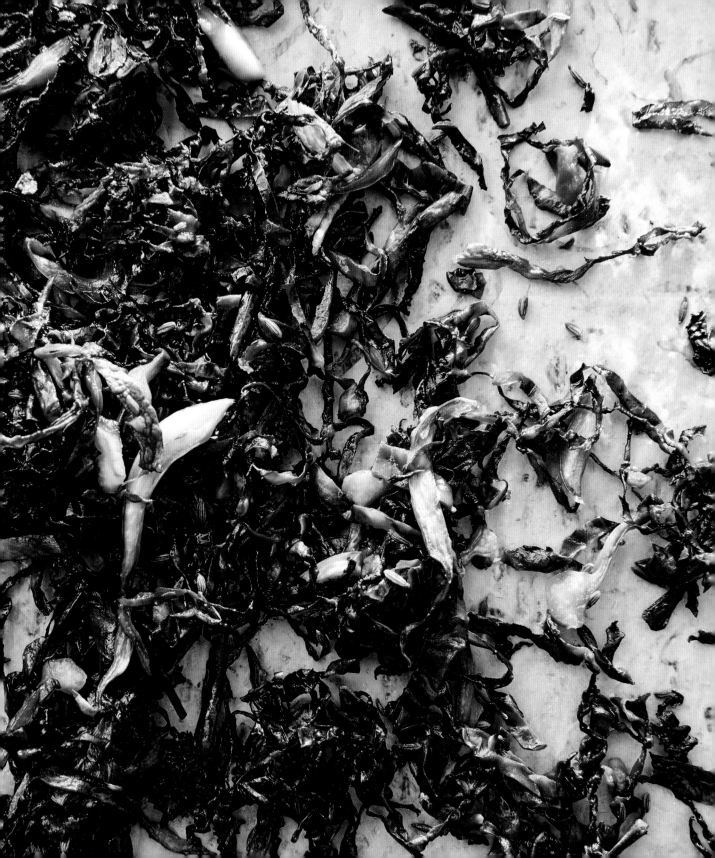

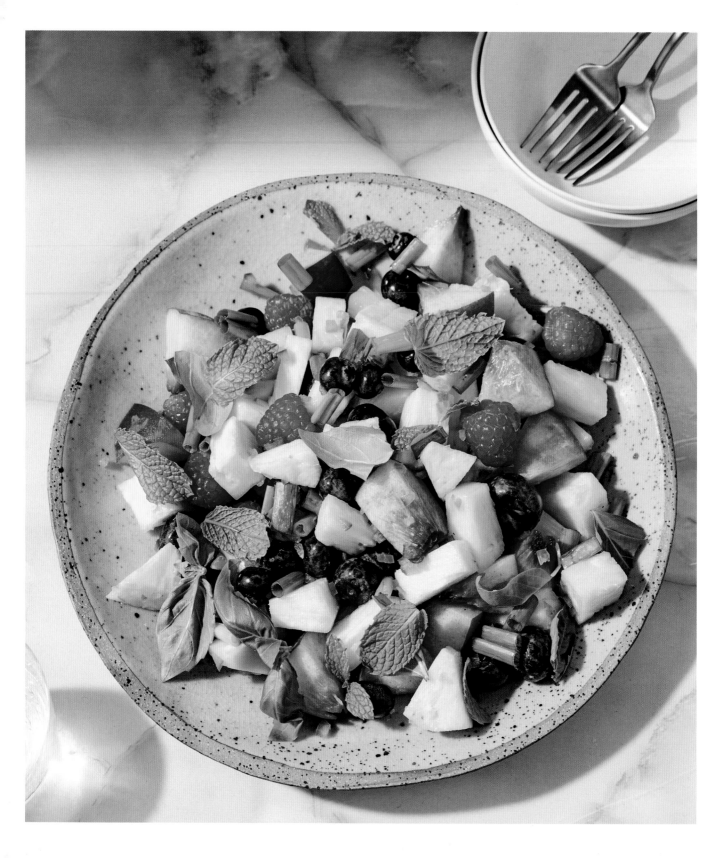

Savory Fruit Salad

MAKES 4 SERVINGS

This colorful, big-flavored salad adds pop to almost anything: tacos, grilled meats, burgers, and roasted tofu, just to name a few. Chop the fruit more finely, and it becomes a delicious salsa for dipping. The jalapeño and herbs in this recipe are optional, but I highly recommend using both if you have them around.

3 cups chopped fruit (such as pineapple, mango, berries, peaches, nectarines, or a combination; ½–¾-inch chunks)

1 scallion, trimmed and chopped

1 tablespoon finely chopped jalapeño pepper (optional)

2 teaspoons lime juice

¼ teaspoon kosher salt

¼ cup roughly chopped or torn herbs (such as cilantro, mint, tarragon, and/or basil; optional)

Combine the fruit, scallion, and jalapeño, if using, in a medium bowl. Stir in the lime juice and salt. Let sit for 5 to 30 minutes. Gently fold in the herbs, if using, and serve immediately.

Quick Cukes

Refrigerate leftovers for up to 3 days. They'll just get more pickle-y!

4 Persian (mini) cucumbers, sliced ¼ inch thick (about 3 cups)

¼ cup rice vinegar

1 teaspoon kosher salt

¼ teaspoon sugar

Put the cucumber slices in a wide shallow dish. (A bowl works, too, but the cucumbers soak up the seasoning more uniformly in an even layer.) Add the vinegar, salt, and sugar and toss gently. Let sit at room temperature for at least 10 minutes and up to 30 minutes, tossing every 10 minutes. If not serving immediately, transfer to an airtight container and store in the refrigerator.

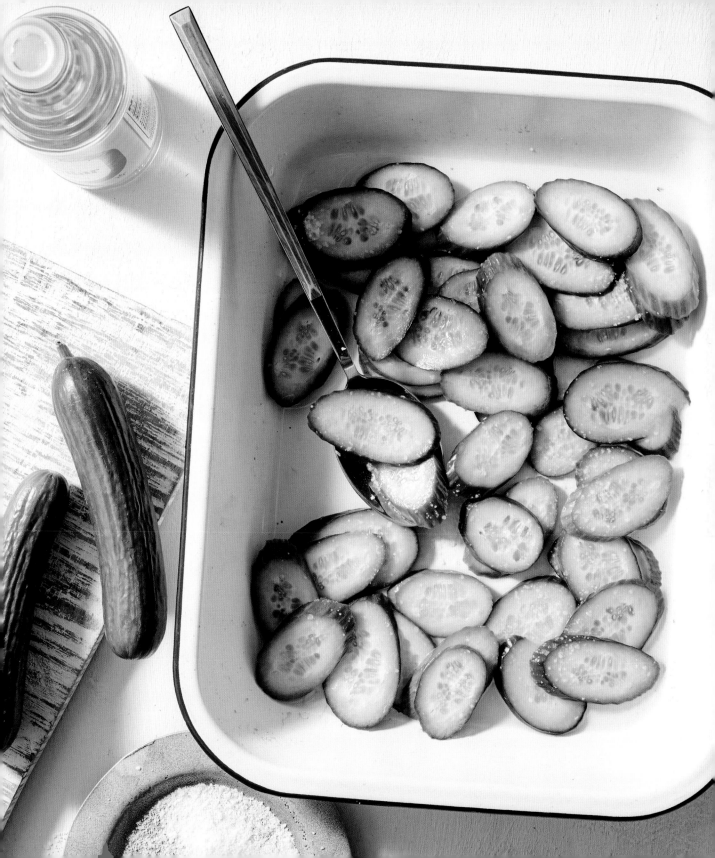

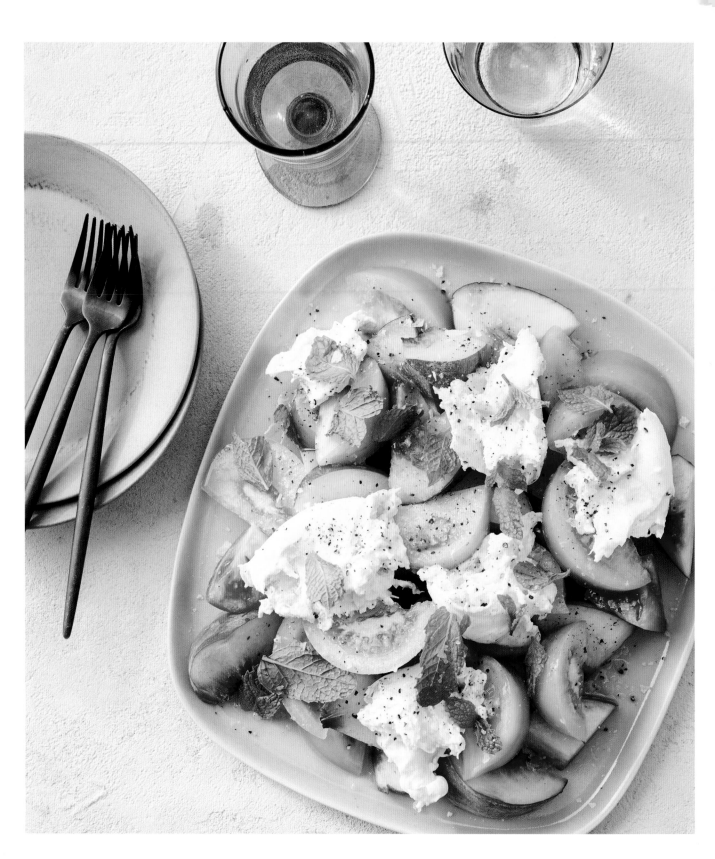

Caprese-ish Salad

A traditional Caprese salad is sliced tomato served with fresh mozzarella and basil, drizzled with olive oil. There's nothing wrong with that! But, my favorite ways to play with this Italian classic are by adding summer fruit to the mix, subbing ultra-creamy burrata for the mozzarella, and replacing the basil with mint. This is one of those dishes where you don't need specific amounts for the olive oil (or salt). My best direction is to be generous.

1 large (or 2 medium) tomatoes, cut into large chunks

2 ripe (but not mushy) peaches or nectarines, pitted and cut into large chunks

Olive oil, for drizzling

Flaky sea salt to taste

4 ounces burrata

Freshly ground black pepper to taste

¼–½ cup roughly chopped mint

Put the tomatoes and fruit on a serving plate, in mostly a single layer (it's fine if there's some overlap). Drizzle with olive oil and sprinkle with flaky sea salt. Tear the burrata into pieces and scatter on top of the tomatoes and fruit. Drizzle with more olive oil, sprinkle with more salt, and top with several grinds of black pepper and the mint.

Quinoa Pilaf

MAKES 4 SERVINGS

Sure, you can just cook quinoa in water. But adding onion (two types!) and substituting vegetable broth for the water gives this simple dish a lot more flavor. Serve it as a side or as the base for a burrito bowl. Leftovers make a terrific salad addition.

1 tablespoon olive oil

¼ cup chopped shallot

1 cup quinoa, rinsed if necessary according to the package directions

2 cups vegetable broth

½ teaspoon kosher salt

1 scallion, trimmed and chopped

1. Heat the olive oil in a small pot over medium heat. Add the shallot and cook until beginning to soften, 2 to 3 minutes. Stir in the quinoa. Add the broth and salt. Bring the mixture to a boil, lower the heat to medium-low, cover, and simmer until all the liquid is absorbed, 15 to 20 minutes. Remove from the heat.

2. Add the scallion to the pot (do not stir), cover again, and let sit for 5 minutes before serving.

PERFECTLY ACCEPTABLE STORE-BOUGHT SIDES

Just heat (if necessary) and serve.

- Frozen sweet potato fries
- Frozen peas
- Frozen corn
- Cornichons or other pickles
- Polenta in a tube
- Canned refried beans

- Applesauce
- Frozen mini spanikopitas
- Flatbread or naan
- Frozen dumplings
- Microwaveable bags of rice or other grains

Index

Note: Page numbers in *italics* indicate illustrations.

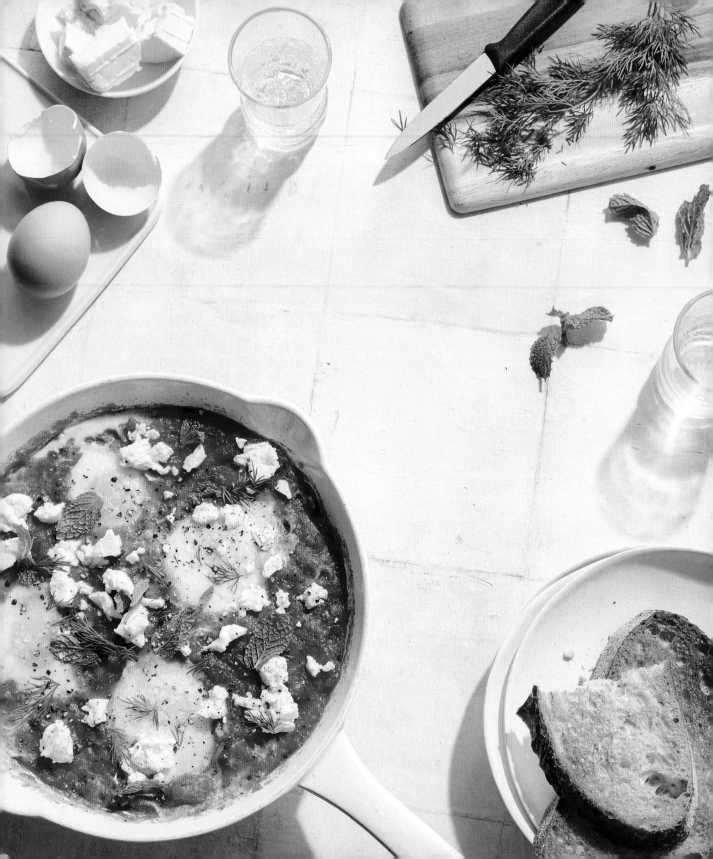